THE BODY AT WAR

AN

INQUIRY

INTO

THE CAUSES AND EFFECTS

OF

THE VARIOLÆ VACCINÆ,

A DISEASE

DISCOVERED IN SOME OF THE WESTERN COUNTIES OF ENGLAND,

PARTICULARLY

GLOUCESTERSHIRE,

AND KNOWN BY THE NAME OF

THE COW POX.

———

BY EDWARD JENNER, M.D. F.R.S. &c.

———

The birth of modern immunology as Jenner reports that a cowpox innoculation can protect one from deadly smallpox.

JOHN M. DWYER

THE BODY
AT WAR

UNWIN

HYMAN

London   Sydney   Wellington

First published in Great Britain by the Trade Division of Unwin
Hyman Limited, 1988.
© John Dwyer 1988

UNWIN HYMAN LIMITED
15–17 Broadwick Street
London WIV IFP

Allen & Unwin Australia Pty Ltd
8 Napier Street, North Sydney, NSW 2060 Australia

Allen & Unwin New Zealand Ltd with the Port Nicholson Press
60 Cambridge Terrace, Wellington, New Zealand

ISBN 0 04 320225 X
A CIP catalogue record is available from The British Library

Printed in Singapore by Kim Hup Lee Printing

Contents

Introduction

W RITERS of books nearly always thank their families profusely in the introduction. So common is the practice that when an author fails to do it, one must suspect that there is no family to thank. If I ever thought such dedications were politic rather than deserved, the writing of this book has taught me otherwise. When one is fully occupied by a demanding career, finding time to write a book is very difficult. While for the author the writing may be a labour of love, for his family it is a demonstration of love, for the time that is normally shared with them is given to writing. For two years my family have lived with the great excuse: 'I must work on the book'. To my wife Catherine and my children Justin, Gabrielle and Christopher, then, my love and sincerest thanks for letting me produce this work.

Grateful as I am to my family, the book is not dedicated to them; it must be dedicated to my patients. For thirty years the sick and the weak have been teaching me how healthy and strong is the human spirit. I specialise in caring for people with chronic diseases. Their courage, patience and ability to structure quality into a life that at first glance has only quantity, is inspiring. I feel privileged to have been able to work in the field of immunology with such patients. Many of their stories are told in the pages that follow. This is therefore their book. Finally, I must thank Boehringer Ingelheim for permission to use their wonderful electron microscope photographs coloured by a computer. They allow us to look at the body at war.

John M. Dwyer
1988

Prologue

I MAGINE that you could stroll with me through a country fairground in Gloucester, England, in the summer of 1794. Here we are, not far to the northwest of London, and naturally we are intensely curious as we take our first close look at our cousins of 200 years ago. Our first impressions are less favorable than we might have expected. To be frank, our ancestors could do with a good bath and some eau de cologne. They are smaller than the average person in our own time, and many look sickly, even malnourished. We look at the faces, study the body gestures and peer into the eyes of these people as we try to learn something about their spirit.

We are struck by their poor complexions. At first we wonder if 60 to 70 per cent of these people have had bad acne, judging by all those scarred, disfigured faces.

In a side paddock, an uproarious competition is under way. Urged on by the crowd, a group of milkmaids is racing against the clock to fill buckets with fresh milk, squeezing with gusto on the udders of protesting cows. The eager young faces of these excited, energetic girls are beautiful; they have fair complexions and the disfigurements noted earlier among the general throng are not noticeable here. Why is it, we ask, that these girls have such beautiful skin?

This question has been exercising the mind of Dr Edward Jenner, a doctor in Gloucestershire, for many years. Jenner's eye for beauty, his skills in observation and his deductive mind combine for a great medical discovery that will answer this question and save millions of people not only from disfigurement but from premature death.

To understand better what has been going on in Jenner's mind, we need to leave the merriment of the fair and travel just two miles to the south to meet one of Dr Jenner's patients. Twelve-year-old Billy Smythe is healthy enough, although he could do with a little more meat on his bones. He does not look much different from the other farm children who help their parents work the squire's land. However, if you look closely at Billy, you will notice that there is a slightly unnatural glow about his face. If you were to inquire, he would admit that he does not feel 100 per cent well.

All day long he has been aware of a headache and a few back pains but has told himself they are not worth worrying about, especially when you think of what happened to cousin Emily. Two weeks ago to the very day, she was playing in his house and seemed full of strength and good humor, even dancing around the kitchen table with him while his father played the fiddle. She had a rather long coughing fit after the dancing, but she certainly had not seemed sick. But now he has heard she is 'deathly sick'.

Emily died six days after her fever started. Billy lasted only two days longer.

Poor Emily, poor Billy. Just like millions of frail humans before them, they fell victim to a tiny brick-shaped foe they would never see. Billy's cousin Emily delivered him into the hands of the enemy. When she coughed over him, millions of the tiny invaders were propelled swirling into the air around Billy's face. Only breath was needed to vacuum into his lungs and thence his bloodstream tiny organisms that would destroy him. They took up residence in his liver and lymph glands, multiplied again and again inside his own cells, only to burst forth to invade the lining of his blood vessels and his skin. Fevers and muscle aches racked his tortured body. Blisters appeared on his skin to give way to deep, pus-filled ulcers, from which the infectious agent jumped to lie on clothes, on bed linen and even in the dust on the floor. In these places it awaited a new victim. Those infected by this ruthless enemy became so weak so quickly that other enemies could jump into lungs and produce a pneumonia, causing the victim slowly to suffocate.

Not everybody engaged in this life-and-death struggle with the unseen enemy lost the battle. Some won, lived to tell the tale and fought further battles with more enemies. Their scarred faces proclaimed their victory over the enemy that came to be known as the smallpox virus.

With this background, we can understand why Jenner was so fascinated with the exceptional resistance to smallpox displayed by many milkmaids. They did not have to fight and perhaps lose the battle with this disease and as a result many stood out from the crowd as beauties.

Jenner had correctly surmised that the reason why the milkmaids did not contract smallpox had something to do with the disease that they *did* get. The cows of the day frequently suffered from weeping ulcers on their udders and milkmaids handling these infected parts contracted a not very prolonged or serious illness popularly known as 'cowpox'. A 'pox' in those days was anything that caused discrete ulcerated sores on the skin. Jenner did not know why, but observed that infection with cowpox, a minimally disfiguring condition, offered protection against smallpox.

After much professional and public debate he convinced the people in his area to let him scratch into the skin of children who had not had smallpox some of the material he harvested from the cows' ulcers. He had heard about the process of inoculation, that is, the introduction into the healthy body, usually the skin, of material obtained from a patient with a disease to try to protect one from that disease. A widely travelled Englishwoman, Lady Mary Wortley Montagu, had brought back from the Middle East tales of dangerous customs practised by the Turks and many others in the region that appeared to protect many from smallpox. In fact, we know that the Chinese as early as the fifth century BC were practising inoculation.

For centuries medical men, from physicians to magicians, had known that the crusted scab that formed over a healing smallpox ulcer on the skin could be protective. Unfortunately, it could also kill. If this dry crust was scratched into the skin (in China it was inhaled into the lungs) one of two things would happen to a patient who had never had a smallpox infection. An ugly ulcer might form at the site of the inoculation and the patient might suffer from fevers, headache and general malaise for a few days and then recover splendid health, protected from small-pox forever. On the other hand, the results of the inoculation might lead to a full-blown attack of smallpox with scarring or death. (Given the danger associated with the procedure, it is an interesting comment on the sexist nature of Turkey in the sixteenth century that fathers insisted on their daughters being inoculated to protect their beauty.)

To comprehend why so many people went ahead and took the risk involved in such inoculation, one has to understand the odds that were being faced. In many areas 20 per cent of the patients would actually contract smallpox from the inoculation itself, but without it the figure for smallpox victims frequently exceeded 75 per cent. Of the latter group, at least 60 per cent could be expected to die.

In all ancient medicine nothing was more revered than the property of the 'pox dust'. Physicians of all persuasions harvested it diligently and stored it as if it were gold. Unlike the majority of ancient medications, this one really worked.

A few years ago I was invited to visit a number of countries in West Africa by the United States Agency for International Development to advise on a number of matters. Unable to walk away from the problems that I encountered on that first visit, I have returned on many occasions since to work on a number of projects.

On one visit to Bamako, the capital city of Mali, I was invited to attend a large meeting of the Malian Medical Society organised for no other reason than to allow the country's minister of health to talk tribal physicians into surrendering their smallpox dust to health authorities.

The World Health Organisation had masterminded a military offensive against smallpox and as a result of worldwide vaccination efforts, had been able to declare that smallpox was defeated. Vaccination procedures could stop. Two potential sources for the reintroduction of this disease remain, however. Some modern laboratories have live virus stored away for research efforts, and some thousands of traditional doctors in Africa and elsewhere have tons of pox dust in which, sleeping quietly but full of virility, are billions of smallpox viruses.

After some debate it was clear that the traditional doctors would not do as they were asked. Smallpox had been here forever and would be here forever and nothing would make them surrender their most powerful medicine. The west African landscape remains covered with biological timebombs.

Without any knowledge that there were micro-organisms that could cause disease, Dr Jenner nevertheless reasoned that cowpox disease (remember that there was no concept of infection) changed one's body so that smallpox could not occur. That is why the milkmaids and many farmers who contracted cowpox were spared from smallpox. To honor Jenner's pioneering work with cowpox (the technical name for which is *vaccinia*) we call vaccines all those materials that when injected into the body produce protection from a specific illness. The procedure for introducing these materials into the body is known as vaccination.

What exactly happened when Dr Jenner scratched the protective pus into the backside of that no doubt protesting young man all those years ago? How was the child's immune system stimulated and armed with weapons that could kill the smallpox virus? How does knowledge of such mechanisms relate to problems we still encounter today, such as eczema, AIDS, poison ivy, cancer, lefthandedness, sensitivity to bee stings, disorders in pregnancy and bone marrow transplants? We are about to explore the answers to these and other questions.

Today most people are interested in how their body works and perhaps even more interested in why it may not work. This is a very healthy attitude. But too much of what is presented as authoritative is just plain wrong. A recent irresponsible statement in a tabloid reported that a clinic in the west of the United States could cure cancer in AIDS victims by the daily administration of caffeine enemas. Desperate people, seeking hope as much as cure, flock to such clinics, only to be robbed before they die.

Most medical publications for lay people, even if correct, are so patronising that the simplifications offered must ultimately be unsatisfying to any intelligent reader who wants to understand *why*. It is with this understanding that this book has been written. While it may help people to enjoy better health, its primary purpose is to inform and illustrate how entertaining and even fascinating the study of the body's workings can be.

With this in mind I will not insult the reader with oversimplification and avoidance of complex details; even the 'mumbo jumbo' that is the terminology of our science will be included. I want to piece together for you one of the most, if not the most, fascinating of all biological jigsaw puzzles and help you find the excitement that I feel you will enjoy when you understand and say, 'Isn't that incredible!'

Our exploration of immunology, of course, must not be slow, tedious and unrewarding. This is not in any way a textbook; rather, my intention is to model this book on the symphonies of Sibelius. As the climax of the symphony arrives, fragments of selfcontained melody come together and suddenly such a flood of luscious melody is released that the heart sings and the soul stirs. While I cannot guarantee that anyone reading this book will enjoy such an experience, I am building my 'symphony' with fragments that will lead us to that sustained melody that is a full understanding of the role of the immune system in daily life.

In any area from allergies to arthritis, from transplantation to viral disease, from T cells to bereavement, the immunologist is involved. I want to show you the excitement that is immunology, the future that is immunology, and make you familiar with that complex but approachable system in whose integrity rests the body's ability to fight so much disease.

PART 1 THE WAR AND THE WARRIORS

1 | Why we need an immune system

IN the fall of 1972, I met an intelligent and worried mother. She told a distressing tale, as puzzling as it was intriguing. Now twenty-eight years of age, she had given birth to three children. The first, a boy, had been perfectly well and developed normally until he was thirteen months old. At that time the young family to which he belonged lived in rural Illinois. When the baby developed his first bout of high fever and irritability, his mother was not unduly concerned; she did not panic when their family doctor took a few hours to come to the house. However, the physician soon recognised that this baby's condition was worrisome: the child was toxic. Alarmed, he arranged for his admission to the nearest hospital which was a good fifty miles from his home.

Meningitis was suspected and then confirmed when streptococcal bacteria of a particular type known as *pneumococcus* were found in the child's spinal fluid. Despite massive doses of appropriate antibiotics, he died twelve hours after admission. An autopsy revealed overwhelming sepsis but no clues as to why this previously healthy child should have become sick and died within twenty-four hours. A tragedy of course, lots of unanswered questions certainly, but, consoled the family doctor, 'These things happen occasionally, bacteria can be deadly. You are young and time and your future children will help ease this pain.'

The next baby born to this couple was a girl who arrived a year after the loss of their first child. Indeed, it was true that time and this beautiful infant did ease that earlier pain, for a while, at least. She was in perfect health and when she was fifteen months old, the family moved to Detroit. When, out of the blue, the child developed the onset of a high fever and listlessness, the now sensitised parents immediately rushed her to the emergency room of a university hospital.

3

She was admitted for observation and her condition rapidly deteriorated. Meningitis was diagnosed, together with pneumonia. The parents must have felt desperate as the all-too-easily-remembered scenario unfolded before them yet again. The same bacteria that had killed their son were found in their daughter's spinal fluid. Again, antibiotics were administered in large doses but were useless against the rapidly multiplying bacteria. Once more, these parents lost their baby within twenty-four hours of the onset of the illness. An autopsy was performed but showed no obvious abnormalities; the baby had simply been overwhelmed by the virulent organisms.

Another consulting physician in another hospital office did his best to answer the parents' anguished questions. How could this have happened to two babies, both appearing to be so healthy in their first year of life? 'It may be coincidence,' said the Detroit pediatrician, 'but it is also possible that there is a genetic defect in your children. Perhaps your babies do not have normal immune systems. They certainly seem to have been unable to present any defense with which to fight these invading bacteria.'

After much anguish, the parents decided on a third attempt at parenthood. A second beautiful and healthy baby girl entered their lives. When this most precious of children was nine months of age, the mother brought her to my clinic and told me the story.

'I know you are going to say the baby looks normal and has had no serious problem and therefore there is nothing to worry about at this stage, but this was true of my other children as well,' she said. 'Please take my baby and find out if she does have a weakness that will stop her from fighting bacteria. Don't let this baby be taken away from me.'

Needless to say, all of us in the clinic were moved by this story and the anguish that this woman was clearly experiencing. She had read extensively and knew that she wanted all the defense mechanisms that act in concert to constitute our 'immune system' checked for hidden, even subtle imperfections.

To the best of our ability we obliged. We contacted the hospitals where the first two children had died. No help was obtained from Illinois, but Detroit told us that they had in retrospect checked the second baby's serum to determine if normal amounts of antibodies (bacteria-fighting chemicals that we will discuss in detail a little later) had been present in normal amounts. No abnormalities were found.

We tested this third baby's blood and secretions for antibodies. We immunised the child with a new vaccine against pneumococcal bacteria. We challenged her white blood cells in our test tubes and in every test that we performed, the baby appeared to be perfectly normal.

Six weeks later the mother, holding her baby close to her, heard the words she wanted to hear from this immunologist: 'I don't know what was wrong with the babies that you lost, but this little one is in perfect condition and has responded well to the new vaccine that we gave her. I am confident that her immune system is working well. Please put the past behind you, relax and enjoy her.'

Four months later, the mother called to tell me that this baby was dead. The news from this anguished mother devastated me more than any other professional loss.

The story of the third loss had been identical to that of the other two, with an instantly panicking mother failing to save her child, despite immediate and competent medical attention.

I have begun my introduction of immunology at this low point for a number of reasons. Firstly, the cases we have discussed allow one to emphasise the lethal potential of the microbial enemies with which we are all constantly battling. Indeed, every day many people, for various reasons, are overwhelmed by infections and die within twenty-four hours. These cases which so baffled us in 1972 also illustrate how rapidly this youngest of clinical specialities is moving. For today, presented with such a story, a correct diagnosis would immediately be suspected, readily established and rapid therapy provided.

The three children described could not make certain types of anti-bodies needed to help defend them from streptococcal bacteria. The word 'immune' is derived from the Latin word for 'protection'. The immune system is a protective apparatus that defends us from that moment when we begin to move down the birth canal to that equally dramatic moment when we need no further biological help. It seems to me logical to begin discussing immunity by explaining from what exactly we need protection. The body's answer appears to be 'everything'. We human beings recognise our bodies as sacrosanct, and do not allow anything foreign to remain in their microenvironment. However, the immediate and correct implication from that statement is that we have a way of knowing the differences between the millions of components that make up our own special body (self) and anything else (non-self). The ability to make this distinction represents the essence of the biological miracle of immunity. We must therefore explore the mechanisms by which the body manages this most demanding of tasks.

Non-self can be divided into two categories that represent problems of very different magnitude. Non-self can be passive; that is, the invading foreignness might not be actively dangerous at all and it certainly will not actively attack us. A splinter in the finger and even someone else's transplanted kidney come into this category. Our body will vigorously reject them both; useful in the case of the splinter, not so good with the kidney.

On the other hand, many examples of the non-self that our immune system encounters are very dangerous indeed, as we have already illustrated. The best examples from this category include the viruses, fungi, bacteria and parasites that invade and will kill us if we do not kill them. In such cases, urgent action is necessary. Often we are dealing with an adaptable and in that sense 'intelligent' foe that knows its immunology. For example, many viruses can deliberately induce changes in our body that will suppress our immune system's capacity to fight.

One further enemy engages our immune system and therefore needs discussing. This one comes from within. Just as personality can change under various influences so that we may no longer equate the person we see today with the one we knew ten years ago, so organic parts of the self can change in such a way that they are no longer recognisable as self. This biological equivalent to the change in personality is known as cancer. A woman with cancer in her breast has changed. The cells that may kill her are very like normal breast cells but there is a subtle and potentially lethal difference. These cancer cells, now out of control, were derived from normal breast tissue. If she (via her immune system) does not kill them, she may die because of what these genuinely malignant cells can do to normal tissues.

As we will explore in detail in a later chapter, the available evidence strongly suggests that in many cases of cancer our immune system efficiently recognises the departure of these cells' behavior and appearance from the normality of self and consequently destroys them. In a number of situations in which certain types of cancer take hold, it appears that the immune system might have failed to realise what was going on and in this sense has let us down by exposing us to the ravages that will follow.

Throughout this book the term *antigen* is used to refer to anything in our body that is not self. Our sophisticated defense mechanisms do such a remarkable job on a day-to-day basis that, for most of us, antigens that enter our body are rapidly handled without their presence disturbing our health at all.

As we have said, some antigens are downright hostile while others, though perhaps painful (such as splinters) are harmless. Before we meet the dangerous antigens that challenge our immune system, i.e., the living microbial organisms that infect us and damage one or more parts of us, producing disease, there is one basic biological unit we must discuss in detail, otherwise all that follows will be unintelligible. That basic unit is the cell.

The cell is the basis of all living organisms, from plants to people. Cells are three-dimensional structures, spherical to cuboidal in shape and made up of walls called membranes that house an array of complicated internal machinery. Imagine that you have blown up a red balloon not with air but with water. Having distended the balloon you now drop a few small pieces of wood into the fluid inside the balloon before sealing

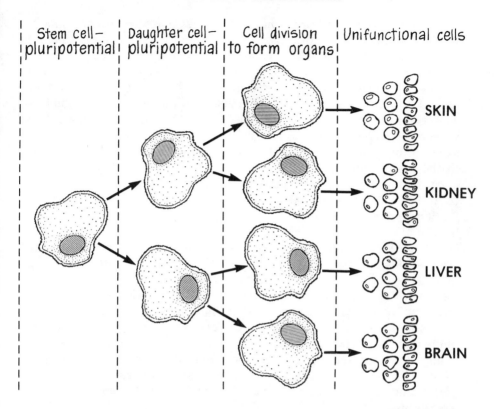

Stem cell—pluripotential | Daughter cell—pluripotential | Cell division to form organs | Unifunctional cells

SKIN

KIDNEY

LIVER

BRAIN

the mouthpiece securely. Such an arrangement gives you a crude mental image of a living cell; expandable membranes surrounding a fluid space that contains specific and functionally crucial structures. Next, imagine placing twenty such balloons next to each other on the floor. On each, build a column of balloons by balancing twenty on top of each other. You now have a wall of 400 balloons (and a secure job with the Barnum and Bailey circus). Obviously, for such a precarious structure to hold together so that balloons do not bounce down the corridor, discharging their contents onto expensive carpets as their fragile membranes burst, membranes must be glued together so that each touches the balloon above, below and to each side. If this is done, the result is a wall of balloons moving slightly, capable of swinging this way and that as pressures are applied. Now, start walking backwards from this remarkable achievement. As your wall recedes, the individual balloons begin to lose definition; and eventually you will think that you see a solid red wall.

Every tissue and organ in our body is composed in this fashion: billions of balloons glued together to form us. We have balloons of many different colors in our cellular repertoire. Blue balloons may enable us to see, red ones can make urine and purple ones make us feel passionate. In other words, clusters of cells all involved in the one function operate in concert as an organ. There is one fundamental difference, however, between the way that we would build a wall of balloons and the way Nature constructs a wall of cells. Instead of blowing up millions of individual balloons and aligning them neatly as a bricklayer might build a wall, Nature makes cells divide to form two, then four, then eight, then sixteen and so on. Each of us starts as one cell that divides time and time again, in fact almost infinitely, to supply us with all the cells needed for the body's various functions.

At some point the products of cell division begin to change. This controlled differentiation allows the various components of the body machinery to develop and interact. Using this sort of imagery by analogy, look at the back of your hand. Your skin looks like an homogeneous layer. Looking at the same skin with the aid of a microscope is like walking closer to our wall of balloons. When you get close enough, the individual cellular elements become clear. While there is no doubt about the fundamental truth of Alan Sherman's words of wisdom, 'You need your skin to keep your insides in', skin, that most useful of tissues, heats and cools us and acts as a first line of defence to keep micro-organisms out of our body. The oily secretions of the skin, the urine secreted by the kidney, the saliva secreted by the cells of our salivary glands bear witness to the fact that the cells of the different tissues or organs are factories performing some specific service to that mighty cellular conglomeration we call 'us'.

Let us go back to our balloons for a moment. Instead of water and a few pieces of solid wood floating inside our expanded balloon, let's imagine that the fluid is really a collection of raw chemical substances and that some of the pieces of wood are assembly lines on which these chemicals could be lined up in a certain order to produce a new and useful chemical.

Every cell is a factory supplied with raw materials made in other cells and designed for that purpose. In every cell is a physical structure known as the nucleus from which is issued operating instructions that tell a cell exactly what its function is. Stored within each nucleus are all the instructional messages needed to run every section of our body, but in any one cell only one of those instructions has been issued. This fundamental biological concept gave rise to the storyline in the Ira Levin novel *The Boys from Brazil*, which concerns cloning. Theoretically if you can obtain and preserve one cell from any individual you have all the coded material needed to generate all the functions of the entire body.

The production plans for each cell, i.e., the blueprints used in assembling the finished product of a cell, are coded by the genes present in the cell's nucleus. Genes are collections of chemicals that deliver messages.

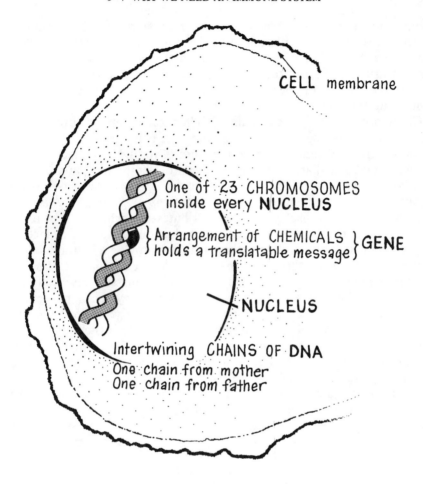

These genetic instructions are actually carried out in the cell's fluid compartment, which is known as cytoplasm.

In one important respect our balloon model for a cell is inadequate. Unless we burst the balloon, the water on the inside will stay inside and the air on the outside will remain there. The membrane of a cell is, however, selectively permeable, i.e., some things can move out of one cell and into another, while essential elements required by a cell are permitted to pass through its membrane. In a very deliberate fashion the membrane of a cell actively controls the movement of various molecules into and out of the cell. Of course, genes control the production of a particular type of membrane for a given cell, so that they can control these environmental fluxes appropriately.

All the genes inside a cell are linked together to form long, intertwining chains known as chromosomes. The genetic material itself is composed of the substance deoxyribonucleic acid, universally known as DNA. Only a small number of genes present in the cell operate at any one time, instructing the cell to do this or that. One can imagine the chaos that would occur otherwise; it certainly would not do to have hair follicles attempting to make blood.

Chromosomes are paired chains of chemicals wrapped around each other. Imagine taking two strands of wire and twisting them around and around each other, and you have a picture of the DNA molecule. Each chromosomal pair that you possess comes from both your parents—one wire from each. Nature, the truly great scientist, constantly experiments, always on the lookout for better combinations of genes. Parents hope that their child will display the best attributes of each, and Nature has seen to it that the miracle of sexual reproduction provides a chance for this to occur. Of course, the mixtures may not provide a better product.

We inherit twenty-three chromosomes from each parent. Imagine forty-six computer programs combined onto one massive disc; only one program can be run at a time. Using this analogy, each program is composed of genes. On the master floppy disc for your life, there are between 300,000 and 400,000 programs that, between them, must produce everything from your most sensitive and intelligent thought to the knee-jerk reflex. We will discuss in detail a group of cells playing the immunology program; cells we call lymphocytes.

We are now ready to examine in some detail those microbial antigens that would kill us without our immune system.

Viruses

I once saw a large neon-lit advertising display in the yard of a car service centre that read, 'Virus is a word used by doctors to mean your guess is as good as mine.'

What motivated the manager to give the world this information remains unknown, but I imagine that this Californian businessman was laid low by a flulike illness. His doctor probably said, 'Not much I can do for you, old man. It's just a virus. Go home, drink a lot of fluids and take it easy for a few days.'

This is admittedly frustrating, but except in the case of very few viruses, it is absolutely accurate advice. Viral infections are essentially private battles fought between the virus and the patient's immune system. Very few effective antiviral agents have been developed so that, except in treating some herpes-like viruses, doctors have very few specific remedies to offer. To date, most success in handling viruses has come from developing vaccines that stop infection in the first place. The inability of the medical profession to do very much about viruses, the difficulty associated with culturing these organisms and the frequently vague symptoms they produce tend to make people think that viruses are strange and mysterious things. This is not entirely true; we know as much about viruses as we do about bacteria.

What are viruses? Looked at dispassionately from a non-human point of view, viruses are very clever and successful life forms (or near-life forms; they cannot survive on their own, as we will see). For a virus to grow and multiply, it must enter into the sacrosanct environment of a specific cell or cells that will become unwilling hosts. Viruses are therefore parasites, living off other organisms.

A virus is composed of genetic material very similar to the DNA in the nucleus of a normal cell. Being composed of genetic material, it carries with it 'messages' — 'instructions' it can give to living but invaded cells, all of which, as we have seen, are factories involved in producing something. The virus instructs the parasitised cell to add to its production repertoire the manufacture of more virus.

A virus invades the cell's computer, which is locked up in its nucleus, and changes its program. As a virus inserts the program into the computer, it instructs the cell to use its own raw materials, normally present for the production of something useful, to put these materials to work to produce more virus. In this way, the simple life form is able to replicate time and time again.

The cells so infected have no alternative but to produce the virus, although they have produced some defense mechanisms to combat the virus. The infected cell dies as it fills up with new viral particles and its membranes burst asunder as the virus explodes through the cell. So released, it simply moves into a nearby uninfected cell and another cycle is repeated. Even if a cell infected with a virus does not die, such damage may be done to the sophisticated control mechanisms that regulate cellular life that a malignancy may develop, i.e., a cancer cell may be born.

In most circumstances, all that stands between us and domination by viruses is our immune system. Its ability to recognise viral infection and deal with it is described later in this book. For now, let us simply emphasise the fact that viruses become part of us, and to destroy them we frequently have to destroy the cell that carries them. If you are unfortunate enough to get hepatitis B, your immune system may have to destroy many of your liver cells to get rid of the virus they are sheltering. If too much of the liver is infected, one may actually destroy oneself (as humans cannot survive without a liver) in attempts to destroy the virus.

Viruses are tiny, they cannot be seen under an ordinary microscope, and this is one of the reasons why their discovery took so long. In fact, these agents were presumed to exist for many years before they were cultured or seen. In 1898 some German scientists were seeking the cause of the disastrous foot-and-mouth disease that affects cattle. They were able to show that disease could be passed from one animal to another using a number of body fluids from infected animals that had been passed through filters known to block the passage of even the smallest bacteria. They called the infectious agent responsible an 'ultramicroscopic filterable virus'. Today, this class of infectious agent is simply called a virus, of which many different types are now known to exist. '*Virus*' is a Latin word meaning a poison that disturbs the soul. Viruses have different shapes and often a biologist looking at a virus can tell much about its properties simply because of its physical characteristics.

It is hard to imagine just how small an individual virus actually is. They range in size from 17 to 300 nanometers: a nanometer is one-millionth of a metre (1 metre = 39.37 inches). As a further illustration, imagine that you put a needle in your skin and allow one drop of blood to emerge. In that drop of blood you would find about five million red blood cells. Each of these cells could very easily house a thousand viruses.

When a virus is reproduced by the cell it has invaded, it is often wrapped in an envelope made of a combination of protein and fatty material and is known as a capsid. This enables many viruses to live undamaged for extended periods of time outside the body. In replicating itself or in designing the envelope in which it will live, the virus programs in a complementary three-dimensional feature enabling it to interact with the specific membrane of the cell it wishes to invade. Quite unwittingly, certain cell membranes carry receptors on their surfaces for certain viruses. It is of great medical significance that viruses are choosy about their hosts. The viruses that cause influenza do not infect kidneys under any circumstances; the herpes viruses that cause so much genital suffering will not cause pneumonia.

Humans are certainly not the only victims of viral infection. Plants, insects and all animals can be infected by viruses. Certain viruses have learned how to invade bacteria, so one could be invaded by a bacterial enemy that has already been infected by a virus. A virus that likes plants, however, likes only plants. Viruses are so specifically designed to invade one cell type that those causing animal diseases rarely infect humans, and vice versa. If one removed the preferred host from the environment, a particular virus would cease to exist. However, we humans have not considered self-annihilation a very good remedy for the problem of viral infections.

How do viruses get into our body? When they are not in their favored hosts, they can be found lying on the floor, attached to a dust particle, resting in the soil or trapped on the fur of animals, etc. To enter our body they must find a break in the skin that might, for instance, follow an accident, the bite of an animal or insect, or the prick of a needle in

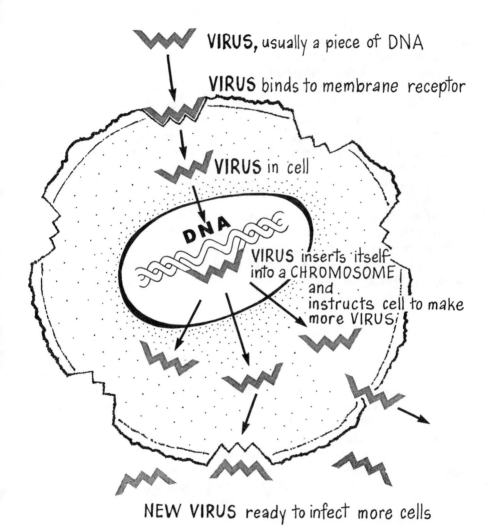

VIRUS, usually a piece of DNA

VIRUS binds to membrane receptor

VIRUS in cell

DNA

VIRUS inserts itself into a CHROMOSOME and instructs cell to make more VIRUS

NEW VIRUS ready to infect more cells

the case of a drug addict. In the last case, infected fluid may be transmitted into our tissues and even our bloodstream. By far the most common way that viruses enter the body, however, is through the mouth. We humans have our mouths open too much of the time for our good, you may say. Besides talking too much and eating too much, we can easily inhale viral particles floating in the air. Millions of viruses leave the nose with a good sneeze; millions enter the air when a room is dusted. Many people frequently put their hands to their faces or place fingers or fingernails into the mouth. Fingers are frequently covered with viruses and hands can become dangerous if unwashed.

Viruses can also leave the body of a strong, immunologically experienced mother and cross the placenta into a fragile inexperienced fetus, doing a great deal of damage; this happens, for example, with the virus that causes German measles. Doctors may inadvertently give their patients viral infections when the instruments they use to peer into or penetrate the body are infected with viruses; even such meticulously sterile operations as corneal transplants that may give someone the gift of sight have occasionally ended in tragedy when the transplanted tissue was infected with viruses.

Now we are dealing with viruses that have learned how to infect and kill the cells of the immune system (the disease AIDS, discussed later), we have been forced to realise once again what dangerous enemies these viruses are. Certainly the last chapter of our battle with these challengers has not yet been written.

Bacteria

I first met Bill in the emergency room of a hospital. This twenty-one-year-old white male was convulsing and sweating profusely as the result of an obvious fever. Having protected his tongue with a mouthguard, stopped his convulsions with Valium injected intravenously and improved his color by administering oxygen, we took a more detailed look at this very sick young man who was unknown to all the regular staff.

Bill was thin, not exactly emaciated but close to it, very dirty and the possessor of a five- to six-day-old beard. The rest of his physical examination revealed three findings of great significance to us. From his arms leaped the bruised, abused and punctured veins of the drug addict, an all-too-familiar sight. More unusual, however, were the sounds coming from his distracted heart, which was beating too rapidly and irregularly. Between the sounds of the rapid opening and closing of those heart valves that ensure the forward movement of blood as the heart contracts was big trouble. Instead of the silence that heralds the smooth onward rushing of the river of life, the sound of a turbulent waterfall vibrated through the stethoscope. As the blood moved from one chamber to the other, irregularities on the normally smooth surfaces of the valves were distorting the powerful jet of.blood in much the same way as a smooth column of water issuing from a partially opened tap may be deviated if a finger is placed in the stream.

The third sign that supplied the pattern-revealing piece of this complicated jigsaw puzzle was found on looking at Bill's hands. Under the nails of three fingers could be seen tiny red spots where miniscule blood vessels had ruptured and spilt their precious cargo into the nail bed.

Adding up all these clues, any medical sleuth could have described the events that had led to Bill's critical condition.

Ten days earlier, he had brought some heroin with money that he had won in an instant lottery game. From a deprived background, unable to work, often in trouble with the law and hopelessly addicted to drugs, Bill must have thought that winning $1000 for a 50c expenditure was a signal from the gods that things were about to change. As it turned out, his good fortune nearly killed him. He bought some 'good stuff' and injected it into himself. Among hard-drug users, the syringe and needles necessary for the injections are often passed from one person to another, to be used time and time again with minimal attempts to keep the apparatus sterile. Often between uses an attempt will be made to rinse out the syringe with tap water, a totally unsatisfactory way to clean the needle. In such needles and syringes, many of the human's greatest enemies, including bacteria, can take hold and multiply.

Bacteria live practically anywhere. In Bill's case, some of the particular bacteria known as streptococcal organisms (strep for short) probably went from the skin of one person into the needle he used for the injection of his 'good stuff'. Once they found themselves injected into his bloodstream, the strep organisms multiplied themselves hundreds of times in twenty-four hours. Blood is an excellent source of both oxygen and glucose, both of which are necessary for bacteria to flourish.

Now, at this point of Bill's story, we must understand more about bacteria, knowledge of which is less than one hundred years old. In fact the first bacteria seen were those that cause leprosy. In a laboratory in Norway, not a country you are likely to link to leprosy, late in the nineteenth century, a certain Dr Hansen looked down his microscope at tissue from a patient with leprosy and saw not one but hundreds of thousands of the little organisms that cause this disease (that, by the way, is why leprosy is often referred to as Hansen's disease).

Bacteria are very different from the viruses we discussed previously, mainly because bacteria are complete life forms. Unlike viruses, they do not need us for their survival. The bacteria that secrete a poison and cause tetanus live just as happily in soil as they do in our bodies. Bacteria consist of one or more cells, each, of course, with a nucleus full of genetic information that tells a bacterium how to be a bacterium. They are much bigger than viruses, although they are still far too small to be seen by the unassisted eye.

Bacteria just eat and divide constantly; they do both better when the conditions are right. We culture bacteria by placing them in a dish in an incubator so that their favorite food source, temperature, humidity and gaseous environment are supplied. Under such conditions, bacteria soon reproduce themselves so effectively that colonies are produced and they can be seen on the surface of the culture dish.

Bacteria can do terrible things to us in at least three ways.

As they multiply in the body, they may secrete poisonous chemicals (toxins) that disturb one or more bodily functions. Some may paralyse our nerves while others block the ability of the cells in our intestinal tract to absorb water into our bodies (think of the terrible diarrhoea caused by the bacteria responsible for cholera).

Bacteria can invade a tissue, e.g., in our lungs they may multiply so quickly that the staggering number of organisms that accumulate may interfere with the function of the organ, causing pneumonia.

When our immune system mounts a vicious attack on the invading bacteria, innocent tissue (us) caught up in the mêlée may be damaged. Such tissue destruction results in an abscess and the chemically digested remains of the bacteria and those parts of our cells inadvertently destroyed are called pus.

Let us get back to Bill who, as you may remember, had just injected some of these creatures into his bloodstream when we left him. The bacteria, of course, were soon racing around his body with no corner inaccessible, because blood goes everywhere.

Now, if you have ever been in Geneva or other places where lakes can easily be studied as they fill up with water racing down from the mountains, you will have noticed that gates are used to control the flow of water. When the gates are fully opened a jet of water spurts through the centre of the opening at great speed but just at the side of that central force are patches of quiet water. That same effect occurs in the heart. Bacteria may have their headlong tumble through the bloodstream stopped when some spin off to the side of the jetstream into the 'quiet' blood. When this happens, the bacteria that find themselves in these less turbulent pools may seed onto the surfaces of the valves of the heart, the gates that control the flow of blood. Here the bacteria may grow in a rich and nutritious atmosphere relatively undisturbed. As they do so, they form colonies, just as they do in our culture dishes. They heap up on the valves and form outgrowths that look a little like the surface of cauliflower; for this reason they are known as vegetations. These vegetations will slowly lead to the destruction of the valves; we can hear this damage in the form of a heart 'murmur' (often in reality a roar). If a disturbance in blood flow is severe enough, the turbulence may often be felt right through the chest wall if the hand is placed flat over the heart. It is just like putting the hand on the cover of a speaker blaring forth loud music.

Bill's heart was in trouble, but the disaster was only beginning. As the heart was no longer able to operate as a smoothly performing pump, some of those bacterial vegetations broke away from the heart valves and joined the bloodstream once more as it raced away from the heart. Now, however, the bacteria were not travelling as single cells, but rather as clumps. One such clump shot up into the brain and, as it passed into some of the tiny blood vessels there to the lefthand side of Bill's cerebral cortex, it became jammed, physically wedged in the tiny artery. Once more the bacteria were able to establish a colony and rapidly grow in the rich sugar-saturated environment of the brain. Eventually they formed a local abscess that damaged the brain tissue itself and led to convulsions and, at a later time (for Bill is still alive at this writing), a paralysis of most of the right side of his body. You will remember that the lefthanded side of the brain controls the righthand side of the body.

In a similar fashion, some of these bacteria broke away from the vegetations on the heart and ended up in vessels under the nail bed where the damage they produced in the blood could be seen through the window that is the cuticle. That is how we discovered what had happened to Bill. He required the services of a cardiac surgeon to replace his damaged heart valves, skilled and prolonged administration of antibiotics and much rehabilitative help. Unfortunately, he is partially paralysed and his intelligence is impaired, but he is alive and no longer addicted to drugs.

The bacterial enemy can live independently, multiply so rapidly and produce so much damage that special antibacterial processes must be generated to supplement the body's defensive mechanisms.

Bacteria have names usually derived from Graeco-Latin words. Most people have heard of *streptococcus* and *staphylococcus*. The *coccus* part of the word, meaning 'chain', refers to the fact that the organism consists of a number of round cells grouped together and clinging to each other in single file, much like a chain. Many other bacterial cells are square or rectangular in shape and when they join together in a single-file fashion they are described as rods. By looking at disease-causing bacteria for different physical properties, bacteriologists can name a particular bug and then physicians can apply treatment (usually antibiotics) known to be effective against this specific organism.

Some of these organisms live in the body's cells where they are significantly protected from antibacterial forces floating around in our bloodstream. (Examples of bacteria that live inside cells include those that produce tuberculosis and leprosy.) As we have mentioned before, bacteria are made up of cells equipped with nuclei so that, as they divide time and time again, they can adapt themselves to fit any environmental circumstances that may come along. When bacteria run into a new antibiotic, genetic information inside the bacterial cells allows them to determine, largely by trial and error, changes in their internal makeup that will allow them to resist its effect. In such cases, the infection will continue after some initial improvement and a breed of resistant bacteria will be launched into the world.

This ability to learn new and nasty tricks is a common feature of rapidly dividing organisms. If we humans become progressively more indolent, in a million years we may look quite different, but the evolutionary changes that may take away lazy legs will occur very, very slowly. On the other hand, bacteria can evolve (that is, significantly change) in very short periods of time. This clearly makes them all the more dangerous for us.

Here is an example of what I mean.

Stewart was in the best of móods and the best of health. He and his girlfriend Helen were happily in love and, after a party, they found themselves alone in Helen's room. They very much wanted to make love, but Helen was hesitant. It was the second day of a heavy period and she was not certain whether he would enjoy sex under these circumstances. However, Stewart brushed her doubts aside. Helen undressed, removed her bloodsoaked tampon and they made love.

The following evening, Stewart was most unwell, with fever and a headache. By midnight he was desperately ill and a worried roommate had rushed him to the emergency room in the hospital, where I was called in to see him.

This strapping young footballer was delirious with a high fever and an abnormally low blood pressure. A red rash covered most of his body and around the edge of the rash the skin was already drying and flaking. The inside of his mouth had red, angry-looking spots on the delicate mucus membranes and he started to vomit uncontrollably. Blood tests revealed that his liver was being damaged and that the particular blood cells needed to help clot his blood were in dangerously low supply.

It was not possible to get a history from Stewart and so, although he was obviously suffering from the effects of a serious infection, we were at a loss to know what organism was causing the problem. We commenced empiric treatment and a battery of diagnostic tests.

When a very concerned Helen arrived in the emergency room, a bright young intern who had been reading some recent literature asked whether she was well, was having a period and had had sex with Stewart recently. When she answered 'yes' to all these questions, we sought her co-operation and cultured some of the menstrual blood in her vagina. We were able to identify 'golden staph', *staphylococcus aureus*, from her blood as well as two dangerous bacterial toxins (poisons) known as types C and F.

Stewart was suffering from a new disease now known as the 'toxic shock' syndrome. The toxins and perhaps some bacteria had passed, perhaps because of a skin abrasion, through his penis into his body and were now attempting to kill him. Stewart's illness might well have saved

Helen from a similar battle as we would have expected her to develop the same syndrome within forty-eight hours. Fortunately, antibiotics were administered in time to protect her.

Toxic shock syndrome is a newly recognised enemy in our chronic battle against bacteria. After much experimentation some *staphylococci* have learned how to produce, given the correct circumstances, potentially fatal chemicals (toxins) that cause the sort of dramatic collapse that Stewart suffered. As far as we know, no bacteria have produced these forces before. The ideal circumstances in which these bacteria can produce these poisons involves the coming together of *staphylococcus aureus* organisms, menstrual blood and tampons, which appear to supply the media on which the bacteria can rapidly grow and secrete their chemicals. As you would imagine, most victims of toxic shock are women, usually under the age of thirty, who absorb these toxins from the vagina.

Warnings about the necessity of being cautious with the use of tampons and the need to change them frequently if they are used are so widespread and commonplace that the occurrence of this problem has become significantly less common in the last couple of years. Certainly, toxic shock syndrome represents an example of how bacteria can change rapidly to give themselves a better chance of survival. Despite the availability of the best in modern medicine, we nearly lost Stewart. A less fit young man could easily have succumbed.

Recently scientists have decided that since bacteria cannot be eradicated, they can perhaps be used to help mankind. A bacterial cell, like any other, is a factory making whatever products its genes tell it to make. We can splice a gene carrying a specific message into a chromosome within a number of bacterial cells and change the production patterns of these cells so that they will produce something specific. Each cell will not produce much, of course, but when cells reproduce as fast as bacteria can, that is no problem. Billions of cells may soon be at work producing something specific for the genius who has mastered them. In such fashion, very large quantities of insulin that can be used by diabetics and growth hormone that can be used by children with stunted growth may be supplied in extremely pure form. Most of the time our immune system can outsmart bacteria, although it is never an easy business.

Fungi

Mary Beth was sixteen when I first saw her. She was in our intensive care unit, her arms heavily bandaged and tied to the frame of the bed. The night before, she had tried to commit suicide by slashing her wrists.

Unlike many wrist slashers, Mary Beth had really meant to kill herself and had very nearly succeeded. She had lost a great deal of blood and was still receiving a blood transfusion. She was wide awake and as I approached she looked at me with eyes that seemed drained of all feeling. Mary Beth had tried to kill herself because she felt herself to be ugly. Hers was an ugliness that made people shiver as they turned away in embarrassment at their obvious inability to hide their shock. What place was there in this world which so venerates beauty for a sixteen-year-old girl with her disfigurements?

Mary Beth's nose was swollen to twice the normal size; a black crust covered most of it. Pus from deep ulcers covered most of her face, and her top lip was swollen and twisted. I had seen a number of people similarly afflicted, suffering from an illness associated with severe breakdown of the immune system.

After receiving indifferent permission to examine the rest of her body, I noticed that she had trouble opening her mouth, but it was clear that the inside of her cheeks and her tongue were covered in a milky white substance. The rest of her body bore isolated ulcers in no particular pattern. Between the upper part of her legs her skin was an angry red color, as was her markedly swollen vulva. A profuse creamy discharge came from her vagina. Mary Beth was the victim of a fungal infection known as *candida albicans*; her disease is called chronic mucocutaneous candidiasis (*muco*=mucus membranes; *cutaneous*=skin). While she could defend herself from bacteria, she had no defense against fungi. Each requires a separate system of defense.

Everyone has come in contact with some fungi. Moulds are fungi; they can grow on a piece of old bread or crawl up a shower curtain. There are literally thousands of fungi, the great majority of which are totally harmless to man. Fungi are another ancient and well-adapted form of life. They always consist of many cells joined together in strands that characteristically branch, sometimes assuming a tree-like structure. In people with depressed immune systems fungal infections of the skin, intestinal tract, lungs and brain are only too frequent. Often fungi are geographically restricted. You will only get certain fungal diseases in certain areas of the world. The fungus that was so troubling Mary Beth had been doing so since she was six weeks old.

This particular fungus, which will be called *candida* for short, is the one your body knows best because everyone grows it in the intestinal tract. Since our bowels are full of bacteria (unavoidable when you think of what we put in our mouth), defense mechanisms have developed to ensure that the bacteria will not only not harm us but also work in our favor. Bacteria make vitamins for us and break down proteins to help us digest and reassimilate the essential nutrients that we eat. But as we have seen, they can get out of hand very easily and may grow so rapidly in our intestinal tract that they swamp our defense mechanisms. To prevent this, a number of strategies are in place. One uses *candida* by allowing it to grow in our intestines and compete with bacteria for essential nutriments. An ecological balance is maintained that prevents excessive growth of either the bacteria or fungus.

It is very common, especially for babies who have antibiotic treatment for, say, a chest or ear infection, to solve one problem while creating another. While clearing up the ear infection, the antibiotics may also kill off the bacteria in the gastrointestinal tract. The result is that fungus can spread up and down the intestinal tract. *Candida* may emerge in the mouth as a white coating on the tongue (commonly referred to as thrush); it may also emerge from the anus and cause discomfort to the skin of that area.

Because of the proximity of the anus to the vagina, it is very common for women to get severe vulval and vaginal infection with this fungus, which flourishes on the moist vaginal lining. For normal people, such an overgrowth causes a superficial infection, with discharge and itchiness being the major complaints. Seldom do our defenses let the fungus penetrate our tissues to cause deep infections. However, if the immune system is deficient, deep tissue infection occurs and serious problems may develop, such as those that affected Mary Beth. Immunologists can now repair the damaged immune systems of patients with this condition, but more of this later. Suffice here to say that Mary Beth fought her disease with courage and today is a happily married working mother.

Parasites

A few years ago I was driving a small, sadly deteriorated Renault through western Senegal en route to the capital, Dakar. On this particular Sunday afternoon, hot and very thirsty, I stopped the vehicle as I approached a tiny village hoping to find some roadside hut selling Coca-Cola. I was out of luck, however, as there were no vendors around and indeed, no one was to be seen around any of the six or eight huts that comprised the hamlet. I stopped the car at the side of the road to drink some very hot mineral water and surveyed a desolate scene. Suddenly, from behind the huts in one of the barren fields, a man came into view leading what turned out to be a procession of thirty or so people walking slowly and in single file across the useless land at the side of the road near where I was parked.

The procession was mainly composed of men. All were wrapped from head to toe in their finest clothes, voluminous robes that enveloped them, despite the relentless heat. Like many of the men in the area, the leader of the procession was very tall and thin. He moved purposefully but slowly, shoulders back and head held high, despite the small, swathed bundle he had in his slightly stretched-out arms. As the column drew nearer I could see tears running down this man's cheeks even though he did not glance in my direction.

Realisation swept over me; I understood that this was a funeral procession. The leader was carrying the body of his young son in his arms and members of the closely knit village were strung out behind him as all proceeded to a shallow grave prepared for the child under a baobab tree. I watched them bury the child, pray and return to their huts again in that same desperately sad and respectful single file fashion.

I went over to the group and learnt more details of this sad event. A five-year-old boy had died that morning after four days of almost non-stop convulsions. He had contracted 'the Pauldism', that is, malaria, which had spread to involve his brain and led to his death. A wandering bush nurse had been consulted three days earlier. He examined the child, who by this stage had bitten his tongue in half, and told the alarmed but hardly surprised community that the child had malaria in the brain and would soon die. Neither he nor anybody could do anything for the child, he assured them as he departed.

During the height of the malaria season in countries such as Senegal, it is not uncommon to have six or more children die from malaria every day in the local hospital. Every year millions succumb to this terrible disease that so sorely tests human defense mechanisms.

Malaria is not caused by viruses or bacteria, nor even by fungi, but by a fourth and major class of microbial enemy — parasites.

Strictly speaking, a parasite is anything that depends on others in one way or another for its ability to survive without contributing to the well-being or the survival of the organism on which it depends. In biological terms, a virus could be considered a parasite. However, when we talk of parasites as enemies we exclude viruses and restrict the discussion, by scientific consensus, to those usually large and complicated organisms that chronically infect humans, particularly in the developing world (unfortunately a major misnomer if there ever was one). Diseases such as malaria and others with exotic names such as trypanosomiasis, leishmania and filiarisis are responsible, quite literally, for most of the human sickness and death in this world. While progress is being made in our ability to handle a number of these diseases, others are more prevalent and more serious than ever. This is particularly true of malaria.

The mosquito that spreads malaria is becoming increasingly resistant to insecticides, the parasite is becoming increasingly resistant to the drugs we use to treat the infection, and governments are becoming increasingly resistant to spending the huge amounts of money needed to control the problem. At least 200 million people are infected with malaria as you read these words. In Africa alone, someone dies of malaria every thirty seconds. That is nearly 3000 people each day, more than a million per year. Malaria is not just a problem for the Third World, however. In the United States about four thousand cases will be treated each year and this number is increasing. International travel exposes many to the parasitic problem of the Third World.

Parasites can be divided into two major groups, the protozoans and the helminths. The protozoan family is made up of many different types of organism, and those that cause malaria belong to this group. 'Helminth' is the technical word for worms; three major forms of worm feast on, or more accurately in, man. Some are roundworms, including the *ascaris* that are common parasites of man. Some worms are flat, like fish, and these flatworms, or tapeworms as they are often called, cause us and our dogs a lot of trouble. *Taenia saginata* is a little worm that we often pick up after a delicious steak tartare. Infestation occurs in all countries where raw or undercooked beef is eaten but it is particularly prevalent in Mexico and South America. The third type of worm is the fluke. This produces the disease schistosomiasis (sometimes called bilharziasis) in 200 million inhabitants of seventy-one countries around the world. The smallest of the worms that infect man may be only two millimetres long, while the largest may be ten metres long.

Protozoans and helminths have an intermediate life cycle, i.e., they live in soil, water or human tissue, but can move into another animal to develop into a form suitable for infecting a human. The malaria parasites mature inside a mosquito until they can infect humans. If the *anopheles* mosquito that spreads malaria could be eradicated, the problem of malaria would be solved.

Malaria is currently the most serious infectious disease problem in the world. When an *anopheles* mosquito comes to feed on human blood, its bite is associated with the injection of its saliva into the body. If the mosquito is infected with malaria parasites, they will be found in the saliva and thus be injected directly into the bloodstream. From this point, they race off to the liver, where they will dive into the cells they find there. The parasites multiply readily until the poor liver cell, acting as an unwilling host, literally bursts with the load of parasites now crowded inside. One parasite in one cell may produce 40,000 replicas of itself. The parasites released after the cell bursts now seek a new abode. Over millions of years they have decided that the inside of the human red blood cell (erythrocyte) is most congenial.

The parasites attach themselves to the membrane of the red cell and burrow inside. As survival of these species is all-important, another round of multiplication occurs inside the red cells. Forty-eight or seventy-two hours after invading red cells (the time interval varies with the different members of the *plasmodium* family) the red cells burst and thousands of parasites seek new red cells to invade.

Now one of the most remarkable survival mechanisms in all Nature takes place; the parasites know that their activities may kill their host, so they must escape into another body before it is too late. Some of them multiply in red cells, but do not rupture them. They wait for the mosquito to return for a second feed.

When these infected cells are sucked back into the belly of the mosquito, the parasites burst from the red cell, develop into mature infecting organisms and migrate into the salivary gland of the intermediate host, ready to start the next heady spin through poor vulnerable humans.

Many humans die of malaria as the organisms produce a severe anemia, destroying too many red cells, and invade the brain or so damage the immune system that other organisms kill the weakened victim. However, most people who have been infected with malaria develop an uneasy truce with the enemy. It does not kill them, they do not kill it and a chronic state of ill health is established. This common chronic form of infection has a disastrous social and economic impact in developing countries.

From the harsh Sahara Desert in the north of Africa to the Kalahari Desert in the country's southern regions, the parasite *trypanosome bruceii* causes one of the most lethal of all diseases—sleeping sickness. In South America a first cousin, *trypanosome cruzi*, infects many millions, causing severe heart and gastrointestinal damage.

The parasite that causes sleeping sickness in Africa is transmitted to humans by several species of tsetse fly. Some forms of the parasite live only in animals and are not directly harmful to humans, though they certainly harm them indirectly. It is regarded as impossible to raise animals for food in more than four million square miles of Africa, simply because of the presence of tsetse flies in the area. All animals living in such an area would die of sleeping sickness.

Infected humans develop definite characteristics. The face assumes a vacant expression, the eyelids continually droop as if burdened with tiredness and the lower lips hang loosely. Arousing the patient and getting his attention becomes progressively more difficult. Patients may eat the food placed in front of them but will not ask for it. They do not initiate any conversation and they become more withdrawn until coma and convulsions signal their entering into the final phases of the illness.

The fly in question picks up the parasites from various animals such as bushbucks. The prarasites then remain expectantly within the fly until a human is bitten. Once transferred under the top layer of the human skin, the parasites, which are strandlike with a moving tail, burrow along under the skin until they burst into the circulation and then head for the heart or particularly the brain. It is the destruction of the brain that leads to the 'sleeping sickness'.

Untreated, the disease is always fatal. Personal protection for travellers in areas where sleeping sickness is a problem cannot be guaranteed, unlike the situation with malaria. However, insect repellents and protective clothing are generally effective, and only 5 per cent of flies in any endemic area are infected with the parasite.

From Chile and Argentina as far north as Mexico, this disease affects more than twelve million South Americans and is the leading cause of heart disease. Twenty-five per cent of the deaths that occur in people aged between twenty-five and forty-four years are attributed to trypanosomiasis. In South America the disease is not transmitted by flies but by little bugs known locally, for good reasons, as assassin bugs. Sometimes they are called 'kissing' bugs. These delightful specimens are all over South America. They prefer to live in animal burrows but will take up residence in cracks and thatches of poorly built country shanties. The bugs come out at night for a blood feed, crawling across the body to find not skin but delicate mucus membrane to bite. They usually find this on a victim's lip where the tough skin gives way to the delicate membranes that pass on into the mouth, where they 'kiss' their victims. The bug often bites the corner of the eye if that is reached first.

The bugs do not inject the parasites into the body as the fly does. Eight to ten days before the blood feast the bugs will have ingested the parasites that have matured in their stomachs to reach their most infectious form. As the tiny bug bites its victims and sucks in some blood it reflexly empties its intestines and drops its fecal material laden with parasites into the wound made by the bite.

There is no satisfactory form of treatment for the American form of the disease.

The debilitating disease known as leishmaniasis or kala-azar is found in parts of Europe, Asia, Africa and south and central America. The leishmania parasites usually live in dogs and rodents and are transmitted to humans by blood-letting sandflies. About 10 per cent of the dogs around the Mediterranean are infected with the organisms, though 90 per cent of the wild gerbils in the southern USSR are infected. Female sandflies suck the parasites into their bellies when feeding on animals and the parasite matures inside its intermediate host. When the sandfly bites a human, the mature parasites are injected into the victim. More than twelve million people are infected with this parasite.

After incubation of three months, a fever, swollen lymph glands, a rapid pulse rate, diarrhoea and cough may develop. The bone marrow is infected and as a result the blood cells usually made here become depleted and anemia and infections follow. Death occurs within three to thirty months in 90 per cent of victims. If caught in time, however, this disease can be adequately treated.

Schistosomiasis (bilharzasia) is the most serious human worm infestation. More than 200 million individuals living between the tropics of Capricorn and Cancer are infected. More than 500,000 people who now live in the USA picked up this disease before taking up residence in that country. The parasites that cause the disease are flukeworms, belonging to the family *Schistosomitidae*. These worms like to live in the veins that drain blood from the intestine to the liver. There they lay their eggs as well as in the bladder, colon, liver itself, lungs and brain. Terrible damage to the host results.

The adult worms are about one to two centimetres in length and they grow in the liver area. The male worms have a central trough running the full length of their body and the female worm lies all day and night within this groove, simultaneously and continuously eating and copulating.

The worms that cause this disease may live for almost thirty years and can lay as many as 3000 eggs per day. The male worm carries the fertilised female upstream against the flow of blood, like a salmon fighting its way upstream to mate. In this way she is able to deposit her eggs in many different places. Some will survive and secrete a substance that damages the surrounding tissues. Now some of these eggs must, for the sake of survival of the worm species, reach the bladder or colon so that they can leave the body in urine and feces. (As we have seen before, parasites must be certain they can get into a new body if they kill the first host.)

The worms deposited with urine and feces in water or soil wait there for their next victim. To survive, they must find and penetrate a specific snail within eight hours of leaving the body. In the snail they multiply and then come out of the snail back into water where they can latch onto and then burrow under any human skin that walks by. No wonder there is so much of this disease in Third World countries where rice crops are fertilised with human feces. This disease is very difficult to control, as it requires massive changes in habits, and no really useful drug for the treatment of the condition is available.

Tapeworms are ribbon-shaped, segmented hermaphrodites. They inhabit the intestinal tract of many vertebrates and unlike many other worms they have no digestive system, so they absorb nutrients along the entire length of their body. On the head is a sucking cup and hooklets are located on the neck. These cups and hooks allow the worm to attach itself firmly to the lining of the intestinal tract. The top part of the worm copulates with the bottom part. The worm can be found in Chile and Africa and is found along the Pacific coast of America, and in northern Florida.

The most dramatic tapeworm infection is diphyllobothriasis, common in Baltic and Scandinavian countries, Japan and Russia. The worm is ingested by fish who pick it up from raw sewage dumped into the sea. If this fish is eaten raw (as it often is) the worm living inside the fish has an ideal opportunity to enter a new host. This worm can grow to be ten metres (thirty-two feet) in length and live for twenty years. Once diagnosed, the infection can be cured. Perhaps the most amazing thing about this infection is that often the human host suffers only minor symptoms of abdominal discomfort and anemia. Occasionally, the worms spontaneously decide to leave the human host. The amazed victim will be psychologically if not physically damaged for some time.

Twenty-five per cent of the world's population, including four million Americans, are infected with a roundworm called *ascariasis*. The adults grow to forty centimetres (fifteen inches) in length. The female releases millions of eggs into the fecal stream in the six to eighteen months of her life at a rate of about 200,000 eggs per day per worm. Once discharged from the body, the eggs may live in soil for almost six years and are taken into their next victim when contaminated food and soil are ingested. In dry, windy climates, eggs can become airborne and inadvertently swallowed. The worms may damage the lungs and the intestinal tract and, although most patients have fewer than fifty worms in their body at any one time, as many as 2000 are not uncommon. Treatment is satisfactory but only education and first-class personal hygiene with adequate toilet facilities will cut down on the attack rate of this troublesome parasite.

Now that we have looked at the enemy, we can turn our attention to the army we have developed for our defense.

2 | The organisation of defense

J UST as modern arsenals are ever changing as the weaponry of a potential enemy becomes more sophisticated, so our immune system has adapted itself many times to counter survival moves made by the microbial world to protect itself. All living things are subject to Nature's rigid laws of natural selection; that is the 'survival of the fittest' principle. Because of the ability of genes to rearrange themselves, no living species is destined to remain locked into a poor design for survival. The pressures they live through (or more importantly fail to live through) suggest experiments for change. Thus, throughout most of time, biological enemies have invested much of their natural energies in efforts to outsmart each other and therefore survive.

Change in the world of Nature can be rapid; in only a few years, many bacteria have become resistant to certain antibiotics, but more often change is very slow by human standards. When we talk of the body's defenses, we mean a system that evolved among developing species over hundreds of millions of years. It was already advanced when humans began their battles with parasites and other enemies some forty to fifty thousand years ago. It is humbling to think that if the history of our planet was condensed into twenty-four hours, and in the last second before the end of that day one was to flash a light beam, that momentary brightness would encompass our time on the planet we now feel we rule.

If we could go back to that primitive time when earthworms first burrowed through the soil and primitive jellyfish lapped at an evolving shoreline, we would find that these simple creatures had already begun the painstaking experiments that would lead .to the assembly of the necessary apparatus for defense. From such humble beginnings developed our modern immune system which, as you will see, is complex. This complexity has been constructed by the constant addition of logical but subtle refinements to the system. The development is analogous to the way that the complexity of a Mahler symphony can be seen to have developed stepwise and logically from the simplest harmonies of the Renaissance madrigal.

The system that we are about to analyse is extraordinarily powerful. Just a few tiny cells from the immune system of a mouse, when injected into an animal of a slightly different strain that has been deliberately made an immunological cripple, can destroy that animal by the fury of the attack that will be launched in just a few days.

Power of this kind brings problems as well as benefits, and much of the necessary complexity of the immune system is generated by the need to *control* these forces within our own bodies. Of all the control mechanisms we have inherited from millennia of experiments, there is one with which our defense system has been most preoccupied. This is a mechanism which should prevent us from making the most awful of immunological mistakes—the attacking of self.

When you are the ever-vigilant protector of the sacrosanct environment of a body, anything foreign that should dare to invade that environment must be rapidly detected and removed. However, finding certain invaders and recognising them as foreign can be very difficult. A major reason for this difficulty is that many invaders look very much like us, not us in the totality of our human form, of course, but in terms of some specific structures that may contribute to the construction of cells. It can be as difficult for our immune system to detect foreignness as it would be for a Caucasian to pick out a particular Chinese interloper at a crowded ceremony in Peking's main square.

Our immune system is up to this task when all is functioning smoothly, but for some of our enemies, looking like us can provide a survival advantage. For example, part of the bacteria that live in our bowel looks very much like bowel itself.

We will approach our immunological arsenal and its uses from the evolutionary point of view, starting with the most primitive system and adding layer upon layer for an overview of the entire system.

Imagine that you are undertaking a review of the security system for an ultra-important, indeed ultra-secret industrial complex, and find that the following system has been devised. All the authorised personnel in the plant and all the goods that have been legitimately brought into the plant display, in an appropriately prominent situation, a vivid identification tag. Anything or anybody that does not display this vivid ID will be regarded as a danger that must be rapidly removed. A system has been perfected in which certain security personnel do nothing but patrol around the complex looking for something amiss.

As the complex is so huge and the area so varied, those doing the screening are specialised, each one educated to spot some specifically suspect situation. For example, a subtle change in a specific program for driving a computer or the rearrangement of a usual packing order for certain stores would be recognised as departures from normal by different teams. These inspectors are not trained to correct the problem they find but rather have the authority and the appropriate signalling capacity to activate various security forces that can physically deal with the problem.

Because different situations may call for different kinds of force, many weapons systems are available to the security forces of the complex, and these can be activated individually. Frequently, however, if the complex is seriously endangered many weapons systems may be called upon simultaneously to ensure the maximum efficiency of the defense effort.

Should a would-be saboteur enter the establishment in the early hours of the morning, our spotters would recognise the likelihood that the saboteur is an intruder and move in closer for a better look using a closed-circuit TV camera that locks on to the suspect and freezes a close-up image of his face on one half of a monitor screen. A computer then runs through all the physical characteristics of the plant's legitimate employees on the other half of the screen, so that with incredible accuracy the physical features of the foreigner and members of the legitimate family are compared. This is the manner in which the intruder will be presented to these vital 'first line of defence' security men who can then be confident that the intruder is just that, and justify the severity of the response that they must initiate.

The moment that they are certain of the seriousness of the situation, these generals must alert the plant 'soldiers' to the danger and direct them to the target. These soldiers are an organisation unto themselves with a hierarchy based on intelligence and training. Certain of them carry receivers allowing them to receive the messages from the inspectors who spotted the infringement. As these men are also highly specialised, an inspector who is trained to recognise the specific problem encountered will activate that specific arm of the response force ideally prepared to handle this particular problem.

A response team will include commandos that will guide a force of variously armed personnel into the battle zone and then urge them to attack. Some of these tactical forces may be more involved in disarming and immobilising than they are in direct killing. So well organised is this team approach that some men have a specific job of cleaning up, removing corpses and other debris from the site of the battle, indeed out of the plant, so that peace can reign again.

Now, as you can imagine, the battle will be brief or protracted, violent or otherwise, depending on the speed with which the intruder is recognised (once established in a secure spot he may be much harder to dislodge) as well as the weaponry he has for resistance and the forces the plant can effectively marshal. One thing is certain; in this highly sophisticated plant bristling with valuable and sensitive equipment, unnecessary force is to be avoided. No use shooting the intruder in the computer room and at the same time permanently damaging the computer. Some innocent bystander damage may have to be tolerated, but one wishes at all times to keep this to a minimum.

As we all know, commandos can get carried away with the glory of the battle and launch a missile when a hand grenade would have been perfectly satisfactory. Therefore, when our inspectors alert the response force, they also pass the same information to the plant's management team, who ultimately have control over matters from that point forward. They must determine the nature and the intensity of the response to be launched for it is their responsibility to ensure appropriateness; enough force to do the job but not more than enough, for excesses may damage the plant unnecessarily.

These management types have also been specifically trained in this business of recognising who is family and who is not, and can thus check the decisionmaking of the team that has sounded the alarm. Via radio communications, these super-managers can control with ultimate authority both the inspectors and the soldiers. In this way, security is maintained and the damage to the plant minimised.

An attack on such an establishment is always a learning process and good management demands that security be strengthened in an area where an attack or infringement was even partially successful. If on two occasions intruders have had some success entering a plant via its large air conditioning ducts, the team that looks after this area must be expanded and equipped for a faster, more powerful response should this previously vulnerable area ever be approached again.

The specialised nature of the work of each of these teams requires personnel who are highly trained. It is not surprising that establishments are available where these skills can be gained and perfected so that on graduation the successful candidates are ready for a particular role in the chain or network of security measures that protect the plant.

The above fanciful sketch, as you will no doubt have guessed, incorporates the major design features of our immune system. The development of the biological system that works on the above principles can now be described.

Tens of millions of years ago, as Nature was designing its first defensive mechanisms, cells were constructed capable of removing large pieces of foreign material that entered the body. The one type of cell responded to all challenges and there were no control mechanisms. For example, a jellyfish could reject a thorn that pierced its flesh in a non-specific fashion. Then, with the passing of many eons, cells that could recognise and attack antigens (anything foreign entering the body) were added to the defensive repertoire of what were still primitive animals in many ways. In further developmental steps control mechanisms evolved. Thus was refined the usually super-efficient system that we are blessed with.

We can examine the evolutionary process in detail by looking at the way in which a tiny human fetus, starting with just a few cells, builds up the complexity of its immune system. Starting after just a few weeks of intra-uterine life, the fetus recapitulates all the evolutionary steps that have gone before, so that each of us during this developmental phase becomes a biological history book.

The thymus gland is the soul of the immune system, and its major products are known as T cells (T for thymus), although their correct biological name is T lymphocytes. The thymus lies right on top of the heart, intimately embracing the great vessels that bring blood into and out of the pump of life. It is in place by the time a human fetus is ten weeks old. Each and every gland develops with the genetic wisdom of the ages displayed in the cells of its biological library, all of which is available to neophyte cells who will learn vital skills during their sojourn in the gland.

In order to attract cells into the thymus gland where they can be educated, the gland secretes chemicals that are irresistibly attractive to certain cells, most of which come from the liver of the fetus. The liver has little to do during fetal life compared to the hugely important role it plays after birth, but it is extremely important in generating pluripotential cells. Through the earliest weeks of life these primitive 'stem' cells, as they are called, leave the liver and spread through the body via the blood vessels. As explained earlier, each of these cells has locked up in its nucleus all the genetic information available to the body as a whole, and the trick that will turn our uneducated 'primitive' stem cell into useful members of the body's machinery involves activating specific genetic programs within a particular cell.

Responding to the thymus, some fetal liver cells begin to fill the empty spaces within the gland. Once they are there, the thymus must make allowance for every one of the billions of individual cells that will be part of the human immune system. The sojourn in the thymus is not easy; 95 per cent of the cells that enter will die.

The cells that survive are brought into physical contact with specific hormones secreted by the thymus gland. These hormones can enter the neophyte cells and, once there, can influence the nucleus and activate T cell potential.

These budding T cells are first taught how to recognise self. To enable self to be recognised, a collection of almost unique proteins is displayed by every cell in our own unique body. This display of 'self' provides the cells of the immune system with a biological mirror into which they can look to simultaneously compare 'self' with foreignness. From the very first development of the immune system, nothing is more important than making sure that we do not attack our own tissues.

The outer membrane of every T cell takes on a specific physical characteristic that complements (in the mirror image sense) those biological trademarks, or 'self' antigens as they are more accurately known, displayed on all our cells.

The concept of 'self' antigen is an important one. At first the term appears to be contradictory; we have previously defined antigen as something foreign to our body and therefore capable of initiating an immunological response. The term, however, is applied to our biological trademarks, because, as we will discuss in our chapter on transplantation, it is these 'self' antigens present on the cells of a donated organ that so irritate the immune system of a transplant recipient. You may also see these same antigens referred to as histocompatibility antigens (*histo*= tissue), another term from transplantation biology. Nature's insistence on us all being immunological individuals makes transplanting organs from one human to another very difficult.

In one sense these 'self' antigens do and must provoke a response from our immune system, though not an aggressive one. T cells can physically interact with our body's own cells. If the interlock is a perfect one, the cell immediately knows that it has definitely recognised self, not foreignness. The recognition of self is an essential preparation for the programming of cells to recognise the enemy.

When an individual T cell leaves the thymus gland, it begins to play its role in protecting the human body. An individual T cell may carry out this task for sixty years. Within the thymus, each T cell is programmed to recognise one and only one foreign thing (for example, a specific part of the measles virus); one T cell one antigen is the rule. As the fragile body has many enemies it is necessary to program among T cells emerging from the thymus the capacity to recognise a million or more quite distinct antigens. The membrane of each T cell possesses a myriad of identical receptors so shaped that the only thing that will fit into them is the specific antigen that T cell is meant to recognise. Every T cell, therefore, has the capacity to recognise simultaneously a component of self and something foreign.

When I said that T cells learn to recognise self, I explained that this was meant in the sense of self as a universally available 'trademark'. Every cell in our body, except our red blood cells, displays the *same* set of characteristic proteins on its surface. The membranes of kidney cells and stomach cells display the flags that proclaim our unique biological nationality. Cells display up to eight major markers that declare us to be uniquely ourselves, plus a myriad of less important markers.

To be accurate, these markers are not absolutely unique to one individual. Nature's permutations and combinations with these markers are finite. Thus we can calculate that something like two people in every 200,000 will be identical. This is very important when it comes to tissue transplantation.

Certain T cells are programmed in the thymus not only to recognise these express markers of self, but also those unique markers that declare that a kidney cell is not a hair cell, which in turn is not a brain cell. In Nature's effort to ensure we recognise *everything* foreign, it has determined that the thymus must generate cells that can recognise *everything*. This means that circulating in the bloodstream, for example, one may find a measles virus–recognising T cell next to one capable of recognising a unique marker on the cells of one's thyroid gland. A T cell programmed to recognise these has the same biological urge to attack the thyroid gland as that displayed by the T cell programmed to attack the measles virus.

This is clearly one of the few mistakes made by the great immunologist in the sky. Because cells circulate in the body that can recognise specific tissues in exactly the same way as other cells can recognise foreignness, humans become potential victims of autoimmunity, that is, the turning of the immune system against self. This occurs relatively frequently. If these self-reactive T cells do what comes naturally, we could end up with diseases such as rheumatoid arthritis, pernicious anemia, diabetes, thyroid disease and a host of other ills. In programming *in* recognition of literally everything on earth, Nature has not been able to program *out* the recognition of our individual tissue characteristics.

Having these potentially autoreactive time bombs inside us means that such cells must be *selectively* controlled. In other words, a cell that would like to attack the lung must be 'told' not to do so; the tissue being recognised, i.e., the lung, is not really the enemy. Remember the controller in our munitions factory who screened the suspicions of others before an attack would occur.

As many individual T cells live for sixty years, these instructions do not have to be repeated frequently and usually all goes well. We live with our potential self attackers by meticulously controlling them. The biological problem yet to be solved, of course, relates to the programming *in* of the recognition of true foreignness while programming *out* the recognition of self. So much genetic information would be required for the task that we would probably need some extra chromosomes if we attempted to develop such a system. This seems to be why Nature has had to settle for a potentially dangerous compromise.

The T cells we have been discussing are ·designed to sound the immunological alarm when the body's integrity is breached. They are known as inducer T cells (a more accurate name than that of helper T cells used until more recent knowledge suggested the refinement). There are, however, four major kinds of T cells.

Why, you may ask, is this so? Why not just have one type that recognises the antigen and kills it without any fuss? The system needs to be more complex for sound evolutionary reasons. To begin with, we need different kinds of T cell to supply us with different kinds of attack mechanism; rejecting a ten metre worm is very different from rejecting an almost undetectably small virus. More importantly, however, the diversity among T cells provides better control mechanisms for the powerful reactions produced in the battle. A network of integrated cells is less dangerous in case one part of the immunological apparatus is deranged. It is better not to have, in this case, all our eggs in the one T-cell basket.

Inducer or alarm-sounding T cells have the special property of alerting other cells and bringing them into the attack. When they sense the presence of the enemy, they can release a chemical they have stored in their cytoplasm called an inter*leuk*in, a hormone-like substance that takes messages from one white blood cell or *leu*cocyte to another. All T cells are members of the leucocyte family, which we will discuss in greater detail below.

Another group of cells is prepared in the thymus to circulate around the body looking for 'their' antigen. When they sense it, however, they must wait for a signal from the inducer T cells giving them permission to attack. The message for these attacking T cells will come in the form of interleukin and other closely related chemicals.

The 'instructions' to these T cells are clear enough: if you sense what you think is the enemy because it fits snugly into your membrane receptor, take a look at 'self' to make sure it is different, and if it is, get ready to pounce. If your assessment of the situation is correct, the inducer T cells will send over some interleukin. Once you react with that chemical, you know you can attack.

We must discuss the actual killing and elimination of invaders in more detail. T cells kill and remove them in one of two ways, although both systems of defense are often brought into battle at the same time.

One particular set of T cells that has the ability to launch an attack against an enemy release chemicals in the form of enzymes (chemicals that facilitate a reaction) around the invader, having been given 'permission' to do so by the inducer T cells. These enzymes bring into the battle cells that are known as macrophages, (from the Greek words *macro* meaning 'big' and *phages*, 'swallow'). These are larger than T cells. Macrophages are activated by T cells and can literally swallow germs and then use the enzymes prepackaged inside them to kill what they have swallowed. They do not always swallow the enemy; sometimes they release chemicals that do a great deal of damage which may be sufficient.

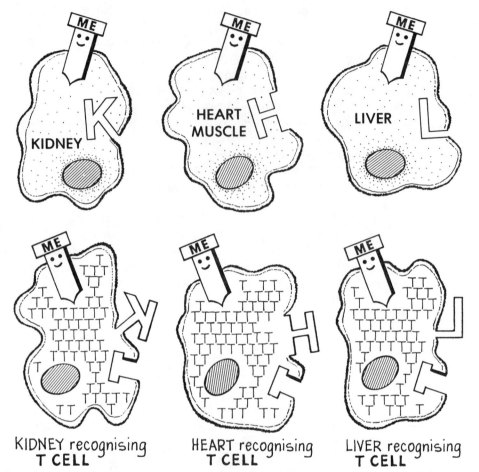

KIDNEY recognising **T CELL**   HEART recognising **T CELL**   LIVER recognising **T CELL**

These **T CELLS** should see **SELF** and NOT ATTACK the cells they recognis

Macrophages are formed in the bone marrow, the space within certain bones that acts as a factory for producing both red and white blood cells. Red cells are red because they have a pigment inside them called hemoglobin which is a red color; white cells are not really white, but colorless. Macrophages start life by circulating in the bloodstream, having been released from the bone marrow in a somewhat immature form, at which stage they are called monocytes. Once they are attracted into the tissues to do battle with an invader, they rapidly mature and are called macrophages.

Other thymus-produced cells known as 'killer' T cells can produce a different form of immunological attack against an invader. Like the cells that call in the macrophages, these wait for a signal delivered by

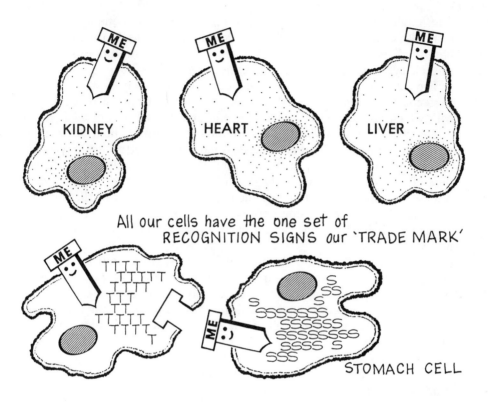

All our cells have the one set of
RECOGNITION SIGNS our 'TRADE MARK'

STOMACH CELL

RECOGNITION OF SELF ANTIGENS

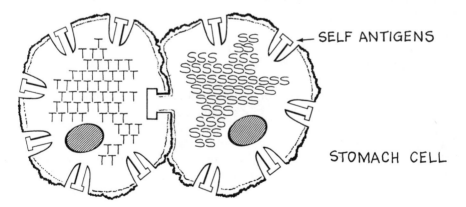

← SELF ANTIGENS

STOMACH CELL

T CELLS have MEMBRANE CONFIGURATION
that permits binding

interleukin before attacking. They move up to an enemy, say for example, a cancer cell, and attach themselves leechlike to the invader or abnormal cell. From a repertoire of more than a hundred poisons stored in their cytoplasm, they secrete chemicals that will kill it.

The immune system is powerful, multifaceted, finely poised between perfection and perfidy. Hence the thymus programs a fourth kind of T cell, which may have the most significant and difficult job of all.

This fourth kind of T cell is the immunoregulatory cell. It determines the appropriateness of the response made to any attack at any given moment; too much destruction launched by the killer cells causes a great deal of unnecessary tissue damage, which must be restricted. Chemicals released by this cell can regulate the extent and efficiency of the immune response. Moreover, the immunoregulatory cells can prevent inappropriate reactions by cells that cannot make the distinction between self and non-self.

Thus we have seen how the thymus gland programs four groups of T cells: inducers that provide our first line of defense, the two groups of inflammation–producing T cells that actually get rid of antigens and the immunoregulatory cells that control the show. I suggest that you reread the security plan analogy if all of the concepts have not fallen comfortably into place.

All this has very recently been confirmed; less than ten years ago, in fact. Thirty years ago, if you had tried to suggest that a T lymphocyte graduated from the thymus with the capacity to recognise an invading antigen you would have been held up to ridicule. That is what happened to the great scientist Paul Ehrlich in 1896 when he drew a picture of a cell that looked remarkably like a T lymphocyte and claimed that this cell, for example, might have the capacity to recognise diphtheria and nothing else.

Paul Ehrlich was seventy years ahead of his time. Even twenty-five years ago, scientists considered lymphocytes to be like soft rubber balls. They claimed that when an antigen (say, a specific type of bacteria) bounced on the wall of one of these immune cells, the indentation so made would remain and the mould obtained from these physical changes could act as a template for the production of specific chemicals that would attack the antigen. This 'template theory' held sway for a long time in immunobiology and it is, of course, now interesting to read that Ehrlich ridiculed it before the turn of the century.

All the T cells we have been discussing are ready for action even before we are born. That very important fact has a lot to do with our ability to survive the hazards of living for nine months in our mother's womb (as you will see in the chapter on the immunology of reproduction). A very important message appears to be given to very young T cells graduating from the thymus during the first weeks of our existence. If the T cells run into anything they recognise before this fetus in which they now circulate is about eighteen weeks old, the thymus programs them to realise that it must be part of the developing baby. After all, tucked up in the mother's womb, one should be, and usually is, sealed away from that hostile and foreign world that is just a couple of inches away. All of our self tissues differentiate by the time we are eighteen weeks old. So a killer cell that is, for example, capable of recognising thyroid tissue, will watch it develop and indeed may bind to it, but during this early phase the cell is told that this is self and must be left alone. In other words, the cell is rendered 'tolerant' to that tissue. Immunoregulatory T cells should keep tolerant that potential killer cell, one that could attack our own cells, throughout our lives.

If by any chance something foreign does cross from mother to baby before our own tissues have fully developed, it is possible that T cells could become tolerant to something that is actually harmful. The classic example is the German measles virus. If that virus crosses the placenta in the first three months of a pregnancy, no reaction will be mounted against the virus. The baby will be born severely infected and severely damaged. If exactly the same virus appears after eighteen weeks of a pregnancy, it will be killed efficiently.

When any of the T cells that we have described see 'their' antigen for the first time, the reaction that follows is called, reasonably enough, a primary immune response. This is somewhat slow as time is needed for specific T cells to meet their antigen and sound the alarm. Quite a few days could pass between the infection and an effective reaction. The second time we encounter such an antigen, however, we are much better prepared. First encounters not only lead to an attack by the invader, they also cause a geometric expansion of the cells with the capacity to recognise the invader. We will probably meet relatively few of the million or more things that we can recognise during our lifetime. This state of heightened preparedness is called immunological memory and is the basis on which all vaccines work; if you get a dose of an invading antigen in a harmless form, you are really prepared for when it enters your body in a dangerous form.

At this point we must introduce a concept that is without doubt the most important in all biology. We humans, and indeed all species, are set to self-destruct. Nature cares for the species with all the devotion and tenderness of a first-class mother, but cares absolutely nothing for the individual. We must die to make way for the young who, ever so slowly, are trying to improve on the older model.

Our thymus gland, for example, works flat out for the first few years of life and then rapidly shuts down production. It leaves us with a lifetime's worth of T cells. After they have gone, so do we.

By the age of sixty to sixty-five in most people, the number and

T CELL   +   VIRUS

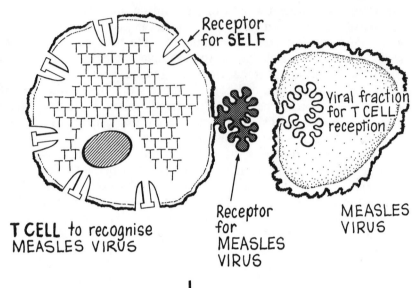

Receptor for **SELF**

Viral fraction for T CELL reception

Receptor for **MEASLES VIRUS**

T CELL to recognise MEASLES VIRUS

MEASLES VIRUS

T CELL ATTACK

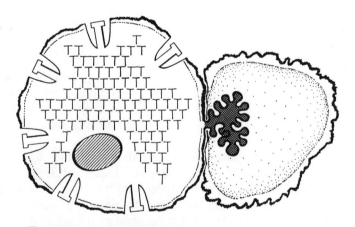

T CELL for MEASLES recognised and bound to MEASLES VIRUS

functional integrity of the T cells in our bodies has diminished. As a result those cancer cells that we destroy with ease at twenty-one become a far more significant problem. Infections become so much more of a problem with older people because of T cell ageing. This means, of course, that we must look after the T cells we possess; they are precious. As you will see when we discuss AIDS, their destruction in adult life leaves us in a hopeless situation. The elusive elixir of youth will need to be capable of rejuvenating T cells.

We have a T cell system composed of regulatory, alarm-sounding and destructive cells that must work perfectly and in harmony on a daily basis to keep us alive. The system itself a very old one; in a primitive, early and tentative phase of development it can be found in an earth-worm. Our sophisticated system is a result of much experimentation over millions of years. The capacity of lymphocytes to recognise, 'learn' by experience, retain memory function and have the self-discipline to act differently and yet appropriately in varying situations make such cells truly wondrous creations of Nature.

T lymphocytes have a home, or more accurately homes, within the body, although for most of their life they travel constantly alongside the blood vessels in smaller 'roads' that carry only the cells of the immune system.

When nine-year-old Christine fell from her bike onto a thorny bush, she sustained minor abrasions to her hands and major bruises to her ego as her accident had resulted from her inability to keep up with her eleven-year-old brother. Her mother washed her hands, placed a kiss and a Bandaid over the small cut on a hand, and life went on. Into that minor wound, however, had entered some bacteria picked up from the thorns and the next day they were making their presence felt. The wound itself was red and a little tender but something was even more noticeable. Christine had a very visible red streak running all the way from her cut hand along her forearm to the crook in her elbow.

In various strategic sites in our body, immune stations have been established called lymph nodes. Vessels in the skin (those that run beside blood vessels) have a fluid circulating in them called lymph. Lymph vessels and lymph itself supply a highway and a transport medium for T cells, and can also pick up an invading antigen that has pierced the skin and transport it via the strong current of lymph flow, to the nearest lymph node. Here the invader is unceremoniously dumped into the middle of the immune army. Under our arms, in our groins, in the crook of our elbow, at the back of our throat (tonsils and adenoids), in our necks and in our bellies (the spleen) are collections of immunological cells grouped together in such a way that they can evaluate anything flowing into the nodes through the lymph vessels whose tributaries branch and then mingle with the cells that populate the gland. In this

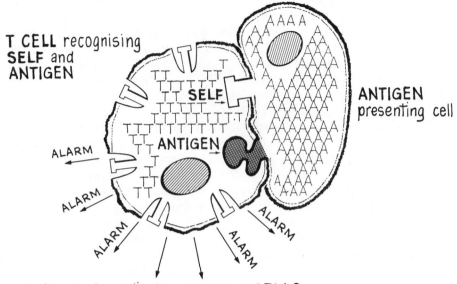

T CELL recognising **SELF** and **ANTIGEN**

SELF

ANTIGEN

ALARM

ALARM

ALARM

ALARM

ALARM

ANTIGEN presenting cell

Chemicals activate **KILLER T CELLS**

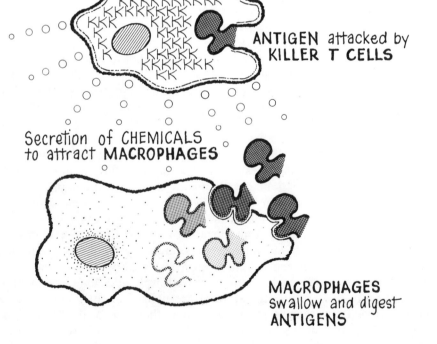

ANTIGEN attacked by **KILLER T CELLS**

Secretion of CHEMICALS to attract **MACROPHAGES**

MACROPHAGES swallow and digest **ANTIGENS**

way, Nature facilitates the recognition of an invading antigen by those few very specific cells that have the necessary recognition capacity.

Sometimes the invading organisms unwillingly being swept along in the lymph vessels secrete toxins that irritate them and sometimes immune cells start to fight an invader even while it is still present in the lymph vessels. In such cases the vessels become inflamed and therefore red and visible. This is called lymphangitis ('itis' always means inflammation). That is why Christine had a red line running up her arm. Once Christine's invaders reached her lymph nodes she recovered quickly, for numerous cells were dispatched to kill the organisms present in her lymph vessels, and anywhere else for that matter.

Lymph nodes, then, are the sites on which Nature prefers to carry out immunological battles; on home ground, so to speak. When this happens, the glands swell. Think of children's swollen neck glands that so often accompany a sore throat.

The glands themselves are wonders of organisational planning, with T cells living in one section of the gland while B cells (which we have yet to discuss) live in an anatomically distinct compartment. Lymphocytes line the edge of the vessel tributaries through which flows lymph and project their recognition antennae for antigen into midstream. In this way viruses etc. running down the river within the lymph gland run a gauntlet of receptors until one or more cells recognises them, grabs them and sounds the alarm. This organisational or anatomical aspect of the immune system is vitally important as it increases our capacity to recognise the presence of antigens.

Some of the lymph vessels and lymph nodes in the chest are very big and large volumes of lymph race through these areas. The biggest vessel of all is called the thoracic duct ('thoracic' means 'chest'). Recently I was called to see a fifteen-year-old boy who had been admitted for surgery to correct a congenital defect in his aorta, the major blood vessel taking blood from the heart. In carrying out the repair, which had been entirely successful, the surgeon had inadvertently nicked the thoracic duct with his scalpel blade. Consequently this vessel was leaking lymph containing many T cells into the patient's chest. So much fluid was accumulating at the base of the lungs that a drain had to be inserted to allow the fluid to escape from the chest cavity and not impair the function of the lungs. But what about all those T cells running away to be lost forever? Billions of vital cells could be lost in a day and a week or more could elapse before those thoracic duct tears healed and the leak stopped.

So important are T cells that we hastily arranged to collect all the draining lymph, race it to my laboratory where we washed the temporarily homeless cells, making sure they remained both viable and sterile, and then infused them back into their original owner. More than 200 billion T cells were replaced over a week in this fashion.

One further piece of T cell biology needs explanation. We are not all born equal when it comes to the T cell system. Within the human family there is a range or spectrum of performance, which means that the ideal of which I have been talking is not always accomplished in a given individual. The consequences of having a second-class T cell system are enormous, as we shall see. While environmental factors can influence the variation basically it is a genetic matter; we inherit a better or worse T cell system as a result of our parents' combining their genetic information.

The B cell system

As we described the T cells system in detail you may have been wondering where 'antibodies' come into the story of immunology. As the term is commonly used you are almost certain to have heard of these proteins. Antibodies enter our discussion at this point and not earlier, as we are approaching the complexity of immunology in an evolutionary sense. The T cell was functioning for 200 million years before the antibodies made their first appearance. Why was there a need to expand our immunological repertoire?

The development and function of the T cell system is impressive but not perfect for the body's defense. T cells do not appear on mucus membranes, such as those lining our throat, intestinal tract and bladder; were we to rely entirely on our T cell system, we would always have to wait until organisms managed to get inside us before the battle proper could commence.

Major problems that literally plagued developing species as they perfected a T cell system came from the world of bacteria. As we have mentioned previously, bacteria can divide (which in biology means multiply) extremely rapidly and spread swiftly through our bodies. They are big in comparision to viruses and may take up so much space that they can severely interfere with an organ's function merely because of their physical presence. Thus, while T cells were handling viruses, parasites and fungi with relative ease, they struggled with most bacteria. Nature, therefore, continually experimented with a separate and new anti-bacterial defense mechanism that, ironically, was broadly understood by men of science long before they knew anything of the far more ancient T cell system.

Over thousands of years of recorded medical history, many doctors have pondered on the mechanisms responsible for immunity. The ancients knew that once a patient had recovered from a specific infectious disease he would usually not have it again, even if he nursed someone who was acutely ill with the disease.

ANTIBODY MOLECULE the product of PLASMA CELLS

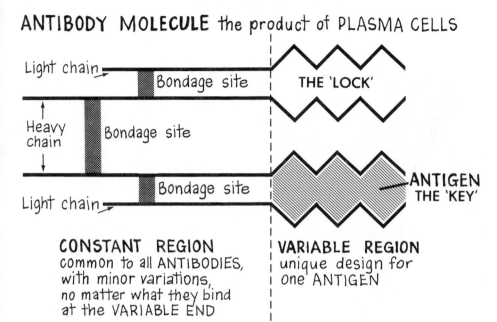

CONSTANT REGION
common to all ANTIBODIES,
with minor variations,
no matter what they bind
at the VARIABLE END

VARIABLE REGION
unique design for
one ANTIGEN

Towards the end of the nineteenth century, scientists discovered that serum contained a protective element. (Serum is blood minus the cells that circulate in it.) This protective substance in serum could be detected only after someone had successfully won a battle with a specific micro-organism. Of course, until scientists had discovered and had actually seen bacteria, they could not have uncovered this fact.

With the discovery of bacteria and the development of the means of growing the organisms in a test tube, experiments could be performed in which such bacteria could be exposed to serum from an individual thought to be immune to that organism. The serum and the organism could be mixed together and the results observed. The ability of something in the serum to damage the bacteria led to the discovery of 'antibodies'.

The system was called, and still is called, for nostalgic reasons, the 'humoral immune system'. Why? Because those early scientists knew a chemical factor in the serum had to be responsible for the antibacterial property and chemicals were so poorly understood that they were collectively referred to as the 'humors'; mysterious things with wonderful properties. Early experiments show that if you heated serum to 56°C the 'humors' vanished, and much interest in the nature of the serum factors responsible led to pioneering experiments that have culminated in the knowledge that those 'humors' are specific proteins popularly known as antibodies, but more correctly call immunoglobulins or gammaglobulins.

A globulin is not, as one student told me, something that runs around the bottom of an Irish garden. A globulin is a protein with some carbohydrate attached to one end.

Immunoglobulins are fascinating molecules, without which we cannot live. They have physical characteristics that make part of them complementary for specific antigens, an idea no doubt modelled on the T cell receptor for antigen. Antibodies are Nature's most exquisite locks into which only one very specific key can fit. As are all the chemicals in our bodies, immunoglobulins are the product of cells. In this case, the cells belong to the lymphocyte family but are B lymphocytes rather than T lymphocytes. The story of how they came to be called B lymphocytes is interesting and instructive.

All birds have a lymph gland-like structure just a little way from their anus or cloaca, known as the 'bursa of Fabricius'. After I had been teaching students about this bursa for many years I decided to find out more about the man Fabricius. He was a leading professor at the University of Padua at the end of the fifteenth century. He was a scientist, lecturer, physician and anatomist who was the first to describe the fact that veins have valves that stop blood flowing in the wrong direction. What this famous man was doing dissecting the backside of birds in 1492 is not easily discovered, but he found the bursa and immortality was his. All birds have a bursa, but what does it do?

As so often happens in science, a series of experiments and chance observations occurring simultaneously in many laboratories have supplied us with the answer to this question. At the end of the 1960s the United States Department of Agriculture was performing experiments to see if chickens could be made to grow faster and hence become more meaty in less than the normal amount of time. Some scientists had the idea of injecting testosterone (male sex hormones) into the embryonic chick before it was hatched to see if this would result in a meatier bird. I guess all the scientists were hoping that the treated chicken embryos would burst forth from their shells beating impressively muscular breasts. The experiments failed, indeed, the little chickens that did come somewhat reluctantly from their eggshells died of overwhelming bacterial infection within a few days of birth. Examination of these animals showed that they had failed to develop the famous but puzzling bursa of Fabricius. It soon became clear from this and other more direct observations that the bursa was the site in birds for the development of those lymphocytes that make antibodies. Birds without a bursa were bereft of bacteria-fighting ability.

This discovery gave rise to the question: Where is the equivalent of the bursa of Fabricius in human beings? It was found to be in the bone marrow. Thus cells that 'learn' how to make antibodies in bone marrow are known as B lymphocytes (or B cells for short).

In the human fetus, stem cells from the liver migrate into the bone marrow in a similar fashion to their movement into the thymus. After birth the bone marrow makes its own stem cells and 'educates' them on the spot.

B cells live only for a few weeks at most, unlike T cells. Consequently the bone marrow must have a production line churning out B cells in great numbers for every day that we live. Each B cell has on its outer membrane almost half a million receptors for one antigen. The biological principle here is similar to that we have described for T cells. These cells wait in the nearest lymph node for the antigen they have been programmed to recognise to come along. If it does, the receptor on the cell membrane which is itself an antibody or immunoglobulin will recognise it. 'Permission' to attack the invading antigen must be provided by a T cell before the binding of an antigen to the surface of a B cell can result in immunological action.

A B cell ordered to attack does so by turning itself into a factory for producing and secreting antibodies. What the cell makes is the antibody or immunoglobulin molecule that trapped the antigen on its membrane, that is, it produces and secretes its surface receptor molecule. When in its full production mode, we call a B cell a 'plasma cell'. Plasma cells can secrete 2000 antibody molecules per second. The B cells are not intended to patrol around the body attacking enemy antigens if they find them, but rather to stay in the lymph nodes and send the antibodies careering around the circulation looking for the enemy.

So our humoral immune system consists of short-lived B cells that recognise antigen, then get permission from a long-lived T cell to attack. In this way, T cells can stop B cells that recognise our own tissues from attacking us, a control mechanism that we discussed when we realised that autoreactive T cells would need to be controlled. B cells then secrete immunoglobulin which goes off to kill the enemy.

Humans make five different kinds of immunoglobulin. These various types are referred to as classes and evolved one by one. With each new model that appears we added something to our infection-fighting repertoire. We always produce our five immunoglobulin molecules in a strict order. By knowing what immunoglobulins are present in any blood sample, we can assess the stage of the response to challenge.

The first antibody to come off the assembly line from inside a plasma cell is called immunoglobulin M or IgM, Nature's first effort at making an antibody. It is not very efficient; it does not last long and it is a biological coward. Five of these antibodies cluster in a pack to watch out for the enemy. This makes the group so big that IgM cannot get into the tissues and simply floats around in the bloodstream. It is therefore limited in its ability to help us fight organisms.

Some primitive species still alive on earth today (some sharks, for example) can only make IgM. However humans cannot survive in our world if they can make only this one primitive form of antibody; occasionally doctors must care for children who are born with their immune capacity limited in this way and they will die if they are not given infusions containing the more important classes of antibody.

When the family doctor gives a six-week-old baby the first shot of diphtheria, pertussis and tetanus vaccine, it stimulates the baby's B cells that can recognise these organisms. Soon IgM antibodies to these agents will appear in the bloodstream, but the baby must go on from there to develop a more sophisticated defense.

The next antibody model to appear after we are challenged by an antigen is called IgD. We know very little about it, as it seems to be secreted in only tiny amounts before plasma cells secrete the next model. It may be important in helping B cells react to T cells.

The third model off the line is IgE (by the way, a T cell tells the plasma cell 'factory when to switch production to a new model). IgE is a fascinating immunoglobulin, the subject of a later chapter of its own, for it is the antibody which, if produced in excess, is responsible for the development of 'allergies'.

Most of the cells that rush to a tissue's defense when it is attacked by an antigen are delivered to the site of the invasion via the bloodstream. As they approach the area under attack the blood vessels dilate, stretching the pores in their wall to a size that is sufficient for the antigen seeking cells to leave the blood vessels and move into the tissues. Unless the blood vessels dilate they will remain trapped within the blood vessels. IgE is specifically designed to release histamine-like agents from specific cells to achieve this purpose. For this reason IgE is often referred to as the immunological gatekeeper.

After the production of IgE, T cells switch production to IgG, the major antibody we humans produce. So important has been this molecule to our defense mechanisms that over the eons it has undergone a number of changes; we can now recognise four subtypes of IgG.

The minor variations in the molecules we produce are very important. They are called, logically enough, IgG1, IgG2, IgG3, IgG4.

Number one protects our tissues from most bacteria, except those that wrap themselves in a coat of sugar. Organisms that can do this include the meningococcus that causes meningitis, the gonococcus causing the sexually transmitted disease gonorrhea and the pneumococcus, responsible for so many problems in the lungs, upper respiratory tract and ears of young and old.

As a response to this defensive move by bacteria, Nature developed IgG2, specifically capable of attacking and destroying these organisms. An inherited lack of the ability to make this particular form of antibody caused the disasters described in Chapter 1 when the young mother lost three children to sugar or polysaccharide–encapsulated bacteria.

IgG3 neutralises certain viruses that race through the bloodstream before diving to safety inside a cell. Once inside a cell, they are immune to the effects of antibodies which are unable to penetrate the cell attacked by the virus.

The fourth type of IgG is a little like IgE, being able to manipulate the chemical-containing cells that open blood vessels; it appears to play an important role in protecting the lower part of our airways.

The fifth and final major class of immunoglobulin to be produced after attack by something foreign is IgA, an antibody that works on our mucus membranes and forms a protective barrier for our 'inner skin'; those delicate membranes that coat our nose, mouth, intestinal tract, bladder and vagina. With the expansion of our antibody repertoire, the body had gained great flexibility in its ability to defend itself.

An antibody is very much like the stylus in an expensive hi-fi set. It can clearly tell the difference between Beethoven's Fifth Symphony and a piece by the Rolling Stones, but just as the music detected by the stylus in a hi-fi set must be amplified if we are to hear how accurately it has tracked the music, antibody detection of an invader must result in amplification of the message so that an all-out attack can be launched.

Just as T cells use monocytes, antibodies have comrades-in-arms that they can call upon. One such comrade is the complement system. This is a fascinating series of eleven chemicals always present in the bloodstream. These can create a chain reaction, each one becoming activated and then activating the next member of the chain. IgM and IgG antibodies, when they bind antigen, can activate the first chemical once they recognise an invader. The activation of these normally inactive chemicals in our bloodstream leads to the amplification of the response that leads to the destruction of the bacteria.

Each activated complement component does something to help eliminate the enemy. Some chemicals dilate blood vessels, others can destroy the membranes of bacterial cells. Most importantly, some of these chemicals attract into the battle a cell we must now discuss. This is known as a granulocyte or polymorphonuclear cell, one that has many shapes and more than one lobe to its nucleus. These cells are extremely important, being our best eaters and destroyers of bacteria.

These cells love nothing better than a sandwich of bacteria 'buttered' with antibodies and complement. This cell does the killing in the B cell system. Obviously it is not much use having the ability to make antibodies if our complement system or our granulocytes are deficient. Clinical immunologists deal with patients who can make antibodies but have problems in these areas, though fortunately such mishaps are rare.

IgA is the 'quiet' member of the family of antibodies. It simply binds antigen and immobilises it so that the complex of IgA and enemy can be moved out of the body as we shed mucin, the viscous fluid that lines our mucus membranes.

Nature knows full well what it has done and realises that humans must make IgM before making IgG, and must make IgG before making IgA. Because of this time delay, special arrangements must be made to help newborn babies who might become infected with bacteria: at that stage of life, humans are so fragile and so many systems are incomplete that bacteria could overcome us if we were not rapidly defended.

Newborn infants, then, are adequately supplied with both IgG and IgA. From the eighteenth week of fetal life, IgG circulating in the mother's serum is allowed to cross the placenta into the baby's bloodstream. This is brilliant, for a baby is likely to be born into the microbial environment to which the mother's immune system has been reacting during the months before delivery. The mother's immune system will therefore be topped up with antibodies against potentially dangerous organisms likely to be encountered by the baby after birth.

The mother can, therefore, passively protect her infant by donating her immunological experience in this fashion. Via this mechanism, babies are born with adult levels of IgG. The amount of antibody they receive will last them approximately three months, usually a satisfactory arrangement, for after the second month of life, babies are capable of making their own IgG efficiently.

This system works better when Nature is left to run it. In many Third World countries, for example, women will take a few hours away from their work to deliver their babies, squatting down and allowing the baby to fall to the ground. After the mother bites the umbilical cord, life can proceed for both. In this situation it is certainly likely that any organisms a baby might encounter will have recently been 'seen' by the mother's immune system.

Modern health care systems have interfered with this in a significant way. When a baby is born in a modern hospital it is likely to encounter organisms that reside in such places and are not present in the general community (nosocomial infections). Consequently, we occasionally face problems because a baby will become infected with a hospital organism. Mother's IgG will not be capable of reacting with this unusual agent.

If a baby is born prematurely, it will receive less of mother's IgG than is desirable and this can increase the risk of infection for such frail infants. Fortunately we now have the ability to 'top up' babies' IgG levels by an intravenous infusion of concentrated commercially available IgG.

What about IgA? Babies are very likely to encounter potentially dangerous organisms that land on their mucus membranes. This is particularly true for the intestinal tract. Nature has solved the dilemma associated with the inability of babies to make IgA by ensuring that breast milk contains abundant amounts. No biological fluid has a higher concentration of IgA than colostrum, the early milk secreted by the breast in the first few days after delivery. Even after milk flow is well established, the fluid remains rich in IgA.

The same principles discussed with IgG apply with IgA. It is very likely that any organisms that will infect the intestinal tract of a baby have recently been experienced by the mother, therefore her IgA is likely to protect her baby. IgA is the remarkable antibody able to survive the passage through the stomach, particularly important to children who must enter the world in less than perfectly hygienic circumstances. This, of course, is why immunologists are anxious to see breast feeding rather than formula feeding emphasised in Third World countries. From an immunological point of view, Nature seems anxious for mothers to breastfeed babies for the first six months of life. After that time, the amount of IgA in breast milk starts to fall quite significantly.

In recent years, doctors have been trying to capitalise on the immunological properties of breast milk by using colostrum and even milk as medicine. Breast milk has been found to be very efficient when used as eye drops, ear drops and nose drops. Indeed, if there was enough of it, giving breast milk to infants with diarrhoeal diseases would probably be very much more commonplace. In many places in Scandianavia, there are milk banks where sufficient human breast milk has been stored for therapeutic purposes.

Apart from IgA and other nutritional wonders, breast milk also contains a number of white blood cells. There are significant numbers of both T and B lymphocytes in breast milk, though it is unclear why this is so. It has been suggested that the presence of foreign cells in the baby's intestinal tract may speed up the maturation of the lymph nodes that line it. Occasionally a mother may breastfeed her baby without knowing that it has been born without T cells; under these circumstances the T cells in the breast milk may recognise the baby as 'foreign' and launch an attack that can be fatal. Normally, of course, the small number of T cells in breast milk would be no match for the baby's fully armed T cell system.

K and NK cells

There are cells circulating in the body and living in lymph nodes that look like lymphocytes but probably have a separate lineage; they do not have enough physical characteristics in common with T or B cells to be grouped in either family. We know more about the function of these cells than we do about their heritage. One group of cells is referred to as K cells or killer cells. These are not to be confused with the T lymphocytes that are capable of killing on their own; rather, these are lymphocyte-like cells with the ability to kill cells that have been coated with antibodies.

This may be particularly important in our defense against cancer; cancer cells cannot be destroyed by antibodies. We make antibodies against a number of cancer cells but they do not seem to be very effective in destroying the malignant, unruly and often invasive cell. However, K cells appear to have the ability to kill many cells coated with antibody. How important these cells are in the human defense system is still not clear, but they probably play a significant role in specific situations.

Perhaps of more interest are cells that again look like lymphocytes but cannot be classified as T or B cells. They are called NK cells; 'natural' killer cells. These have the ability to kill certain organisms and cells apparently without any help from other sections of the immune system at all. They seem to work more efficiently when in the presence of chemicals released by activated T cells.

We have talked about interleukin, which can deliver permissive signals to both T and B cells. Another potent chemical released by T cells is called interferon. This chemical has some anti-viral and anti-cancer properties but also seems to stimulate NK cells to kill virus-infected cells and tumor cells. As we will see later, there seems to be a connection between the performance of NK cells and various psychological factors related to stress. This whole matter will be explored in great detail later in the book.

Well, there you have it. A sophisticated, integrated army that for most of us performs splendidly for seventy years or more. Clearly it is one of the glories of biology.

PART II   TAMING THE WARRIORS

3 | Pregnancy, Nature's version of transplantation

C ATARINA had been married for eleven years when I first met her. As is the case with many young couples, she and her husband had not wanted children immediately. After three years of married life, she had decided to start a family. She stopped taking contraceptive pills and jubilantly informed her husband three months later that she was pregnant. Healthy and relaxed she looked forward to motherhood with intense excitement.

Catarina's first pregnancy lasted ten weeks. She lost the baby easily, with little discomfort, not after a fight with her husband, not after a fall, not even after a horse ride. She was having a dinner party for a few close friends when she felt a trickle of blood down her leg and some crampy pains in her stomach. It was all over very quickly.

She and her husband were bitterly disappointed but not alarmed. Thousands of healthy women have miscarriages. However, three more miscarriages followed. On one occasion she managed to take a pregnancy to twelve weeks but she usually lost her babies between the eighth and tenth week of her pregnancy.

The toll from her disappointments was considerable. She became depressed, she lost weight, she became more introspective. Her husband was as much concerned about his wife as he was about the elusiveness of paternity.

One obstetrician said that perhaps her cervix was too relaxed. He advised her to become pregnant once again, stay in bed for the entire pregnancy, and allow him to put a stitch into her cervix after she became pregnant so that the baby could not possibly fall out. She did all three of these things and lost her fifth fetus after nine weeks. (The obstetrician, by the way, was correct when telling her that some women lose babies because of problems with the cervix, but this was not the cause of Catarina's problems.)

Another doctor speculated that the reason she was losing her babies was that they were abnormal, genetically imperfect. He had often examined miscarried specimens and found them to be abnormal. But it seemed unlikely that five babies in a row should have been rejected for this reason.

When I met Catarina, who was Chilean, she assured me that she could have literally purchased a baby in a matter of weeks for ten thousand dollars in Santiago. However, she ached for her own baby.

Catarina brought her problem to America — to Providence, Rhode Island, to be exact. She had been advised that there was a Chilean-born but naturalised American obstetrician who was interested in women with Catarina's problem. She came, he listened, then he phoned me and said, 'I have Mary's "twin sister" here in the office and want to run a few simple tests. But if the results are normal, will you please check her out?'

I was only too pleased to so promise, as our Chilean-American obstetrician and Mary had aroused my immunological interest in the problem that faces women who spontaneously and repeatedly abort their fetuses.

The 'Mary' of our phone conversation was a twenty-eight-year-old nurse with flaming red Irish hair who had only just delivered, albeit one month prematurely, an otherwise healthy, red-haired girl, the spitting image of her mum. This was her first successful pregnancy; seven previous conceptions had terminated spontaneously. Mary's problem was that she was too close to her husband. Was Catarina's problem also caused by the same strange set of biological circumstances?

One is not long at medical school before learning that a woman has to be close to her male partner to become pregnant. The closeness problem suspected here was clearly not physical.

As it turned out, we were correct with our assumptions about Catarina. She and her husband were third cousins and their histocompatibility profiles were remarkably similar. Before we finish this story, however, we need some more background information.

Lust, love and lymphocytes are inextricably interwoven into the complicated tapestry that determines the survival of the species: we will concentrate here on the role of lymphocytes. As we look in detail at the immunology of conception and pregnancy, we will see that Nature has developed many mechanisms for perfecting and protecting the single most important thing we can do; reproduce ourselves. There is no room for having all your biological eggs in the one basket here.

With orgasm, the woman contracts her vagina to help move the thousands of sperm cells so generously donated by her lover to the mouth of her uterus and, more importantly, to those small canals that run off from each side of the uterus, known as the Fallopian tubes. Conception without orgasm is possible, of course, but more difficult. Hundreds of sperm cells equipped with wickedly vibrating tails swim against the tide to move upstream so that they can enter the Fallopian tubes. The man has therefore impregnated the woman with foreign material. (Note that 'self' is not lying in these Fallopian tubes.) Immunologically those thousands of squirming, pushy sperm cells are just as immunologically abhorrent as would be gonococcal bacteria. Surely the woman will not fail to reject them!

But if the woman does reject those foreign sperm cells, unceremoniously disposing of them, she will never be fertilised and the species will die. She could accept sperm cells that carried genetic information identical or nearly identical to her own, treating them in a privileged way as 'self', but this would not advantage the species; experimentation is Nature's rule. The woman must give a selective advantage to the sperm cells from someone who is very different from her; Nature is indifferent to the fate of cells that look like those of our potential mother. On the other hand, *not* to reject those cells would surely require a suppression of the woman's immune capacity, which would be dangerous. There is no point in getting pregnant and then dying of pneumonia.

The vaginal lining with its rich blood supply is in contact with this foreign seminal fluid and cells for some time. Given that foreign protein to which one is repeatedly exposed should generate an increasingly vigorous response, *why* do women (usually) fail to reject sperm?

Deep in the testicles, cellular 'factories' produce hundreds of thousands of sperm cells, which, when ready, go to the prostate gland. The prostate is part of a man's sexual apparatus.

It produces the enriched support fluid in which the sperm cells are suspended. This seminal fluid has wondrous properties, not the least of which is its ability to block inflammation. It is very largely responsible for blocking an immunological reaction to the sperm cells and other injected proteins that would otherwise provoke an immunological response in the vagina. How it does this is still not perfectly understood, but it seems likely that there are chemicals similar to prostaglandins in the fluid, and we know that these chemicals can stop inflammatory reactions.

After foreign material has been launched into the vagina and blocked any local reaction, using the immunological soothing balm that is seminal fluid, many sperm cells will have made it into the Fallopian tubes. The cells break free from the seminal fluid as they swim upstream in locally produced fluids, for they all wish to penetrate an ovum, the little egg produced by the ovary. Their antigenic (foreign) potential is displayed to the local immune system in the Fallopian tubes and yes, it does react to the challenge. The more foreign the sperm cells, i.e., the greater the genetic difference between the man and woman, the more the potential mother's local immune apparatus is likely to be activated.

However, the immunological response in the Fallopian tubes helps rather than hinders fertilisation. With thousands of invaders, the response made by the woman's immune system is not fast enough to destroy all the cells. All that is needed is for one and only *one* sperm cell to meet the ovum, penetrate its membrane and intertwine its male genes with the female genes therein, in that most loving of embraces that actually sparks life.

The ovum is the ultimate proponent of monogamy. After fertilisation, her outer protective membrane is no longer penetrable; the door is slammed shut. All the unsuccessful candidates are then destroyed and rejected. When this happens, as is usual with any sort of inflammation, there is a degree of local swelling in the Fallopian tubes. As a result, the Fallopian tubes' diameter narrows and the passage of the tiny fertilised egg, which has now become all important and is already beginning to divide, is significantly slowed. This is very important; the fertilised egg might otherwise tumble back down the Fallopian tubes into the vagina and be lost.

Slowing the passage of the fertilised egg is important for another reason. The destination of the fertilised egg is the wall of the uterus (womb), and this organ must have time to get ready for the guest who plans to stay for nine months.

Rats do it differently, but we tumbled on the secrets outlined above in studies of these invaluable partners in our search for scientific knowledge. The rat has a uterus divided by a membrane, into two separate 'wings'. Scientists took rat sperm cells and injected them into one wing of the uterus. The rats experienced an inflammatory reaction only on the injected side proving that sperm was really antigenic and that immune responses could occur in the womb. Subsequently, when the animals were allowed to inject sperm cells naturally and a pregnancy occurred, it always occurred in the wing of the uterus that had been previously stimulated by the scientist's injections. The immunological response in the womb turned out to be a vital part of the mechanism needed to establish a pregnancy.

From the above, it will not surprise you to learn that mice that are deliberately inbred to produce a colony of laboratory animals that are genetically very similar are less successful than are wild strains in their attempts to fertilise each other.

We have already discussed the concept of our biological trademark; protein flags on the surface of every one of our cells that declare each of us to be individual. An individual's membrane 'signature' represents an almost unique creation. We have discussed the fact that we use these markers to help us differentiate 'self' from 'non-self'. Our immunological system reacts to the virus in the throat, compares it with our trademark, realises the difference, and attacks.

When those trademarks of 'self' enter someone else's body, the recipient reacts violently, unless by pure chance they are perfect replicas of that bodies' own markers; a very unlikely occurrence. To a large degree the violence with which we treat other people's cells is graded by the extent to which they differ from ours. At least eight major and very many more minor protein flags are involved in this system. If two people are identical, except for one major flag, the immune reaction provoked will be less intense than if they are totally dissimilar. (This concept is explained in more detail in the chapter on transplantation.)

The more dissimilar the cells of a man and a woman, the better for the genetic mixing we have discussed. We now have the ability to examine in the laboratory cells from a couple in order to determine just how different or similar they are in this histocompatibility (tissue compatibility) sense. When this was done with a number of childless couples without obvious cause for their infertility, where the mother had experienced repeated miscarriages, you may not now be surprised to find that many were genetically closely matched.

When we mixed cells from such couples in a test tube and let them fight it out, we found a very weak response to each other's 'foreignness'; normally, a battle to the death ensues. This is exactly what we found when looking at Mary's and Catarina's problems: each had close genetic compatibility with her husband.

If this is true, however, why did Catarina have to go through twelve weeks of pregnancy before her miscarriage? Well, by dint of a lot of sexual industriousness and the sheer numbers of sperm cells involved, a pregnancy under circumstances of genetic compatibility can occur, if less efficiently than with other couples. But the fact of Catarina's repeated miscarriages suggested that immunological responsiveness was important not only in getting a pregnancy under way, but even more important in maintaining it.

Once that fertilised egg buries itself into the wall of the prepared uterus (implantation) and hooks itself, via the burrowing of its primitive umbilical cord, into the mother's blood supply, the battle for survival is just starting. The baby that looks (genetically) too much like its mother is in trouble all the way.

If you think about it for a moment, you will realise that an established pregnancy is the ultimate transplantation situation. Sitting in its mother's uterus is not a kidney or a heart or a liver, but an *entire human*. Half the genetic complement is its mother's, but the other half is its father's and that is immunologically objectionable. If after the pregnancy, or even during it for that matter (although it's a little hard to arrange) some of the baby's skin is grafted onto mother's skin, it will be promptly rejected: we know this from animal experiments using inbred identical strains that can supply us with a living animal identical to one developing in the uterus. When a baby is born, the mother's blood is full of antibodies against those paternal trademark antigens that the baby now carries and that are dissimilar to her own. In fact, we use donations of such blood to help us type an individual's genetic profile. In this respect a woman who has had six children by six different fathers is a biological treasure, for her blood is full of antibodies to a very broad range of histocompatibility antigens.

It is therefore obvious that we must discuss and then dismiss one of the myths about motherhood and realise that superficial appearances are deceptive. We are always seeing the image of a contented mother with a Mona Lisa smile looking benignly at her swollen abdomen, hands resting lightly on the tumour that she is apparently so willing to accept. Down in the depths her body is trying its best to reject that paternal parasite. It is, however, mysterious to relate, the very fury of her attack on the fetus that allows it to survive. How could a continuous immunological response to a developing fetus protect it, rather than destroy it?

To explore this we must introduce two new characters to the story. One, who is only remotely involved, is that great seventeenth century scientist, Sir Isaac Newton; the other, who is indeed very intimately involved in all of this, is the immunologically intelligent baby.

One winter's day Newton was skating on a frozen pond with a friend and in a jocular fashion, pushed (playfully shoved may be more likely) him away. As he watched his friend slide on the ice, he (Newton) noticed that he went backwards also. On the frictionless ice, his passive friend had displaced Newton as much as Newton had displaced him. Newton raced for a stick, put it on the ice and the two stood toe to toe on either side of this soon-to-be-famous stick of wood. Newton pushed and the two skaters moved away from the stick. As Newton had predicted, the distance they travelled was equal. The harder Newton shoved his friend (who must have been a patient, meek soul), the further they moved away from each other. The distance travelled by both, however, always remained equal. One can imagine Newton racing around the ice, screaming at everyone who would listen, that 'For every action, there is an equal and opposite reaction!' or something close to that.

The weapons of the immune system consist of inflammation-producing cells and regulator cells that control the former, and ensure that any response is appropriate. The *stronger* the immunological attack that is launched, the stronger the dampening influences produced by the immunoregulatory cells.

There is a slight variation on the Newtonian theme in the immune response. If both 'go' and 'stop' signals were equal all the time, nothing would happen. Therefore, the reaction is more like two tug-of-war teams, with one (attack) team having a few more muscle men initially. Soon, however, they lose this advantage when the other (regulatory) team recruits more help and both teams come back to the starting position once again. Both teams are acting simultaneously; the result is only a matter of balance. What we are looking for in our pregnancy story is a balance situation in which the immunological response against the baby gives an advantage to the suppressive forces.

We know that if mother and baby are generally similar, relatively weak suppressive forces are generated, with the result that the mother's immune system continues slowly but persistently to reject her baby.

How is the 'attack team' weakened and the 'regulatory team' strengthened during pregnancy?

The raging of the mother's lymphocytes against the baby is hindered by three major factors that tip the balance in favour of the baby: the mother's powerfully stimulated regulator cells exert a 'go easy' influence on her aggressor cells, the wall the baby has built around itself defends it from aggressor cells and the baby's own immune system helps suppress the mother's T cells that could endanger its survival.

By ten weeks of fetal life, the baby's immune system is beginning to explore the environment in which it finds itself and gets ready for defense. What does it find itself up against? On the outside we have the mother, all love and devotion, knitting bootees, satisfying one-time-only excusable cravings and being thoroughly spoilt because of her ordeal. Inwardly she attacks her child; when she retches in the morning, she is showing her real biological feelings about the growth down below.

The poor little baby must be separated from the mother by a series of membranes constructed to wall it off from an intensely hostile environment. At one point (the placenta), these membranes are organised to allow certain blood elements and maternal nutritional factors to be filtered across to the baby. Unless those membranes are breached, the mother's angry T cells can't get at the baby. If the membrane is destroyed, a miscarriage will result.

Nature, however, supplies babies with an instinctive defense mechanism of their own which helps diminish the danger that is all around. The baby's immune system allows all the young regulatory cells to secrete their suppressor chemicals; as no battle is going on inside the developing baby at the moment, the baby can afford to be immunosuppressed. These chemicals are sent across the placenta into the mother to tame her T cells.

The cells perform their task. This does place the baby at risk of being overwhelmed by an infectious agent should one manage to cross the placental barrier at this vulnerable time. It is more important to worry

The Genetics of Fetal Survival

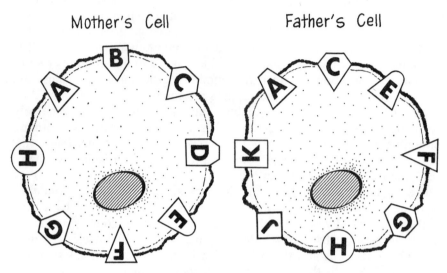

Mother's Cell   Father's Cell

Display of **SELF** ANTIGENS too similar — rejection

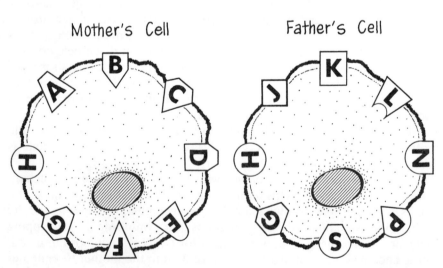

Mother's Cell   Father's Cell

Display of **SELF** ANTIGENS not similar — success

about the mother's aggression, however. Fetal self-help in this fashion may not be enough to save our would-be baby if other mechanisms are not in place, but it may be the additional suppressive force that makes all the difference between survival and rejection.

This survival move on the part of the baby can be of great help to certain mothers. As we will discuss when considering autoimmune diseases, those horrible affairs where our immune system attacks us (for example, in the case of rheumatoid arthritis), the basic defect in such situations is one of regulation. Victims of these diseases lack sufficient regulatory chemicals to block autoaggression. When a woman with such a disease is pregnant, the baby may float enough immunoregulatory substances across the placenta and into the mother to actually suppress the autoaggressive tendencies she has developed which are causing disease. She will bloom during the pregnancy, only to have her problem recur twenty-four hours after she delivers her child.

Another hazard must be faced by male babies. The majority of fetuses spontaneously aborted are male. Mothers can actually be driven to make an extra effort to reject their baby if it is male. Why? Because males proudly display their sex by means of a biological trademark never, of course, displayed on female cells and therefore always foreign to mothers.

Fathers determine the sex of their babies. Their sperm cells may be either female or male, while the mother's eggs carry only female genes. When a father's sperm selects a son, he is sentencing his offspring to an additional immunological hazard.

It is of considerable relevance to the theme of this chapter to learn that women living under considerable stress may experience a moderate to major degree of immunosuppression. The result is that they are less able than usual to attempt rejection of their fetuses. Perhaps it is not surprising, therefore, that in times of stress more male babies are born. This was very well demonstrated during World War II when the birthrate for live males soared. By the way, the male marker makes it slightly more difficult to transplant a male kidney into a women with kidney disease. These concepts and the effects of stress on the immune response are dealt with in detail later.

Pregnancy, the most astonishingly perfect example of adaptation; allows a 'transplanted' body to survive inside an immunocompetent woman. As you can imagine, immunologists are trying to develop the knowledge and skills necessary to apply similar methodology to prevent the rejection of transplanted hearts, lungs, livers, etc., and of course for the treatment of those all-too-common autoimmune diseases.

As we have mentioned earlier, mothers make many antibodies against the paternal antigens possessed by their babies. Antibodies, as we have seen, can cross, and indeed must cross the placenta and enter the baby's circulation if, at the moment of birth, babies are to have some protection from the hoards of bacteria that assail them. Why don't the antibodies directed against fetal tissues harm the baby? It seems that within the placenta is a very clever sponge arrangement. Here are expressed strongly (visibly) a host of paternal antigens. Antibodies heading for the baby will be absorbed by the 'sink' and only good antibodies will cross into the fetus (i.e., those that will not react with the baby's tissues).

The placental unit is also capable of secreting hormone-like agents. Of these the most interesting is known as PAPP (Pregnancy Associated Plasma Protein). PAPP is very important for the maintenance of a normal pregnancy, and, fascinatingly, its release by the placenta occurs only when there is an immune response to the fetus. PAPP seems to amplify the function of those immunological cells that down regulate the aggressor cells. Nature is determined to have a lot of 'fail safe' techniques operating at once to protect her most valued experiment; the unique genetic mixture.

Back now to childless Catarina. We explained all the above to her, and gave her the results of the test we had done on her cells and those of her husband. The degree of genetic similarity between the two fell within the range we were suspicious about. There was a good chance she was successfully rejecting her babies.

Catarina was advised that she had a reasonably good chance of having a baby, if she were willing to take a small dose of a cortisone-like drug throughout her pregnancy. Cortisone can, among numerous other effects, suppress immunological responses. There were minor risks to her and her baby with the approach, but we were confident that they could be handled without too much fuss.

So it proved. I'll bet her son, by the time of this writing, is already a fine horseman.

This is not the approach that would be used now, a few short years later. Work on the problem has progressed rapidly. Women in Catarina's position are being 'immunised' with their husband's tissues before they become pregnant. Injecting cells and extracts from one's husband's tissues into the skin and blood stream on a number of occasions can increase a woman's immunological reactivity to the minor differences that do exist. The result in these early days of this form of research are encouraging. In one series, 78 per cent of women previously unable to complete a pregnancy because of compatibility gave birth to normal children.

4 | Human attempts at transplantation

THIS book celebrates the wonder that is the healthy human body. Arguably the most sophisticated of Nature's creations, our bodies function with a precision, indeed a perfection in no way approached by the most marvellous of man's creations. We are the most intelligent of creatures and can therefore analyse and appreciate the gift that has been given to us to clothe our souls. The same intelligence, however, tells us that we are not perfect. One of our imperfections is youth. Oh, young bodies are close to perfection but they are so often guided by intelligence *sans* wisdom. As a result, beautiful bodies are wrapped around telegraph poles and damaged by inappropriate diets and generally abused in the name of good times and freedom. Would that maternal wisdom, like maternal antibodies, could cross the placenta and top up our young until they could supply their own!

It was lack of wisdom that led two young sisters to abuse their bodies with a poison that brought them to my attention at a time when they were holding onto their lives by the most tenuous of threads. Susan and Marion were fifteen and fourteen years of age respectively at the time. They were schoolgirls who lived on a farm in the north of Connecticut.

These girls should have been healthy, and Nature and their parents had done a good job with them, then they started sniffing gasoline. This is not a rare problem; the sniffing of dangerous aromatic substances from glue to gasoline in order to experience pleasurable release from reality is increasing.

As so often happens, a tangle of circumstances allowed the girls to drift towards their deadly addiction. The family farm was not doing well. Oil prices had soared and this small farming unit was heavily mechanised. Only with the latest in farming machinery could the girls' father make a profit; even with good equipment, he needed to work from dawn to dusk to make ends meet. So it was that, somewhat reluctantly, the girls' mother went back to work in a nearby town as soon as she felt her children were able to look after themselves for an hour or so after school. The girls had four younger siblings, two boys and two girls. They were healthy and not involved with the older girls' problems.

On the property was a large barn in which tractors and other mechanical devices were garaged and it was in this barn that Dad kept his large drums of gasoline. Sue later told me that she remembered having enjoyed the smell of gasoline since she was a child and that the barn had always been a special place for the children, a sort of warm, unreal, refuge for playing and fantasising. Thus I suppose it was not especially surprising that Sue should take the cap off the cans of gasoline housed there to enjoy the aroma that filled the air.

Unfortunately, on one fateful day, she lent over the drum and actually inhaled the aromatic fumes deeply; why she could never tell. She could relate, however, the marvellous effects that the inhalation of these fumes had upon her. It made her feel 'so good'; cares disappeared as worry was displaced with a giggly lightheaded feeling. She inducted Marion into the sniffing club and soon it became their habit to come home each day from school and head straight for the barn and their 'high'. This they were to do for three to four months, and their tired and no doubt preoccupied parents did not begin to suspect that anything was wrong.

The first sign of trouble came when Marion started to bruise easily. The merest bump of thigh against table would lead to a nasty bruise; she became covered in them. In retrospect, the mother was to tell me, she had noticed that both girls had been listless for a couple of weeks before the bruising episodes.

An alarmed mother made an appointment with the family doctor who ordered some blood tests. He told Marion and her mother to come back in four days to discuss the results, but within twenty-four hours he was on the telephone telling them that something very serious had happened to Marion's blood. The doctor explained that the major problem appeared to be an extremely low platelet count.

Platelets are cells produced in the bone marrow which circulate in our bloodstream primarily to help blood to clot efficiently. When a blood vessel is damaged even slightly, the pressure within the vessel associated with blood being pumped so forcefully around the body makes it very likely that some blood can leak from the damaged artery or vein into the tissues. Therefore, no matter how tiny the breach in the vessel it is rapidly plugged so that precious blood cannot escape.

Damaged blood vessels secrete a sticky substance to which platelets adhere. They in turn effectively plug the break, then they activate the clotting factors that are present in blood. A clot occurs around the break in the vessels. This will dissolve slowly but only after the vessel wall has healed itself completely.

Normally we have about 250,000 platelets in every drop of blood. Marion's count was down to 4000. But she had other problems as well; the cells that help antibodies in our fight against bacteria, i.e. the neutrophils, were also much reduced in number. Needless to say, young Marion did not connect this problem to her gasoline sniffing. A very concerned mother and family doctor had the child seen immediately by a hematologist, an expert in blood diseases. After listening to the story and examining the child, the specialist immediately admitted Marion to hospital.

That same night after her shower, an alarmed Susan displayed a number of developing bruises to her incredulous parents.

Sue joined her sister in hospital, for the abnormalities in her blood were identical to Marion's. Given two children with the same problem, their physicians very soon started looking for some shared exposure to a toxic substance to explain the girls' condition. In so doing, they unravelled the gasoline-sniffing story. Gasoline fumes have long been known to have the potential to destroy many of the cells we find circulating in our bloodsteam so the cause of their abnormalities was obvious, even if the prognosis was not.

The gasoline vapors, containing dangerous chemicals, had been inhaled into the girls' lungs, whence they were readily absorbed into their bloodstream. Once in the bloodstream they were easily delivered to the girls' bone marrow. The delicate mechanisms responsible for the education of so many vital cells in the bone marrow were poisoned. Sometimes with supportive measures such as blood and platelet transfusions, time can be bought to allow the marrow to recover from the toxic effects of the vapors. Sometimes hormones may help in the process. None of these approaches helped Sue and Marion and the girls were seriously ill when I first met them.

When it became clear that they would die before their bone marrow could recover (presuming it could ever recover), recovery would obviously require a successful bone marrow transplant operation, i.e. a gift of marrow cells from a healthy person. Once transplanted into the bloodstream of the girls, these cells could dive into their marrow spaces and repair the damage.

Both mother and father volunteered instantly but just as quickly we assured them that neither would be suitable. The girls needed marrow cells that would not be distinguished from their own marrow cells. Why? Because if the cells were different, one of two consequences, both fatal, would occur.

If the children's own T cells were intact (and they were; the gasoline had not affected them), non-identical marrow cells would be ruthlessly

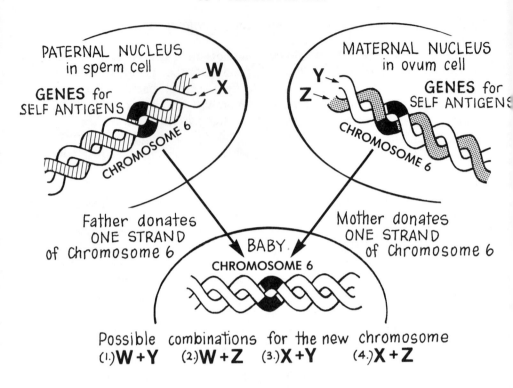

Possible combinations for the new chromosome
(1.)W + Y (2.)W + Z (3.)X + Y (4.)X + Z

attacked and no engraftment (take) of the donor cells would occur. If we suppressed the children's T cells with drugs (which we could do, but it would be dangerous) the non-identical cells that had been transplanted might kill the children. Marrow contains many T cells that actually reside there and exert a major influence on the production of all the blood cells made in the marrow, not just the B cells that make antibodies. These marrow T cells could 'recognise' the children as foreign and 'reject' them, attacking many tissues simultaneously.

The disease that would result is for obvious reasons called graft versus host disease. The donated T cells would roam around the body attacking the skin, brain, liver and intestinal tract first, but eventually all organs would fall before their attack. A death from graft versus host disease is a miserable one. No, the girls had to have identical marrow or they were doomed.

Their parents had each been responsible for donating 50 per cent of the genetic information that had been translated into a Sue and a Marion. The reason for the 50 per cent split is important. All genetic information is encoded on chromosomes; think of songs (genes) on a tape (chromosome). Chromosomes are in fact paired structures (two strips of magnetic tape wrapped around each other). When a germ cell is

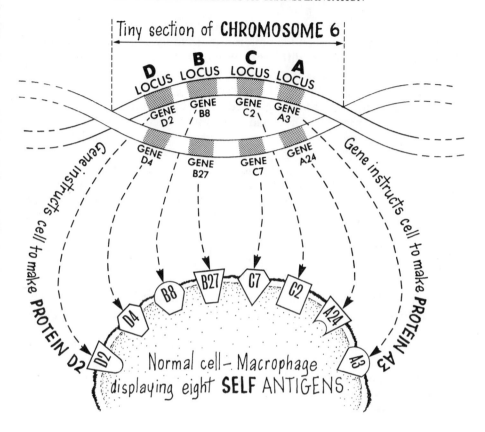

formed, i.e. a sperm cell or ovum, only one of the two entwined chromosomes (50 per cent) is carried along. For this reason the children could not be identical, in a genetic sense, to either their mother or their father.

In the nucleus of each human cell are twenty-three pairs of chromosomes. Each pair is recognisably different from the other and so geneticists can identify each of them. They are given numbers to identify the first twenty-two pairs (1–22) while the twenty-third pair, which determine the sex of an individual, are, reasonably enough, referred to as 'sex chromosomes'. When it comes time to form a new human being, one chromosome from each of the twenty-three pairs will be donated to the new offspring by both mother and father.

If each of the mother's twenty-three genetic programs (chromosomes) is split into two equal lots called W and X and the father's into two equal lots called Y and Z, it is obvious that, for any given chromosomal pair, all the couple's children must consist of one of four possible genetic formulae: WY, WZ, XY or XZ. With each pregnancy there is an equal

chance that any of the formulae will turn up for each pair of chromosomes. Thus three consecutive children in a family could have the same
formula or could all be different. While that would be a matter of
chance, what is certain is that if there are five children in a family any
particular genetic pairing must be repeated at least once.

Sue and Marion were being plied with blood, steroids, platelets,
antibiotics and prayers. They had one hope: each needs to find one
sibling with the same genetically programmed tissue profile as herself.

The genes for the eight major biological trademarks' (self or histocompatibility antigens) and a myriad minor ones that pepper the surface
of our cells are located on chromosome pair number six. Susan and
Marion needed a sibling who had inherited the same combination of
maternal and paternal histocompatibility genes as themselves.

As things turned out they were indeed fortunate children; each had a
sibling who was a perfect match. Susan's brother Paul was ten years old,
Marion's was baby Rachel, only four years old. There were ethical
considerations, of course, in using the sisters' siblings at such a young
age but the parents, physicians and the Institute's Ethics Committee
agreed to the propriety of the desperate measures being made to save
the girls.

The donor children were anesthetised and large bore needles were
inserted into their hipbones to allow the precious marrow to be extracted.
The cells obtained were washed, diluted and injected intravenously into
the two desperately ill children. After injection the marrow cells race
around in the circulation but spill out of the blood as they pass through
the marrow to take up their new residence in the previously poisoned
spaces. It never ceases to amaze me how cells can know exactly where
they want to live, but the homing instincts of all sorts of cells that live in
specialised tissues within our body are unfailing.

After this form of transplantation it is always a touch and go situation
for the two weeks before the marrow starts to produce new cells but,
happy to report, these girls recovered completely and their siblings came
to no harm as a result of their generosity. The family is now united as
never before and the two young ladies are much wiser. I doubt that they
will ever have so much as a puff of a marijuana cigarette.

Now, except for the case of identical twins, the situation we have just
described is about as good as one will get in the transplantation business.
While you work within a family grouping, variations in the histocompatibility (or transplantation) antigens are limited; once you break away
from the family group the odds of two people sitting next to each other
on an aeroplane being identical in this sense are about 200,000 to 1.
Consequently if you are in hospital waiting for a kidney transplant, your
chances of having your 'mate' brought into the emergency room almost
dead and having a card in his wallet saying 'In case of my death please

use my organs' is very slim indeed.

Before discussing organ transplantation let us consider in a little more detail these biological trademarks that make transplantation so difficult.

Anyone who is to have a transplant is 'tissue typed', that is, his biological trademarks, present as membrane-bound proteins, are characterised. With the help of computers and sera from women who have had many babies there are now bottles of testing material that contain antibodies to all the different trademarks in our community. These markers are given names. On chromosome number six there are four places (loci) where the genes that produce these things reside. The loci are called A, B, C, and D. In the human community there are very many different genes that could occupy each loci. Only one gene will be present at each loci in any individual, but remember that chromosomes are paired and therefore there will be eight genes in all involved in the major histocompatibility system.

This means humans inherit one A, B, C, and D set from each parent.

We can place human cells from a potential organ donor or recipient into tiny wells in a plastic tray and then suspend them in a small amount of fluid. We can then add to each well a drop of antibody known to react with a particular histocompatibility antigen. As we usually use human white blood cells (leucocytes) for the task, the system is often referred to as the HLA or *h*uman *l*eucocyte *a*ntigen system. If the added antibodies bind to the cells in a well, then the cells will clump together and fall to the bottom where they will be observed as a small white dot. One of the eight antigens has therefore been 'typed'. So you may end up with a profile that looks like this: Mr Smith's HLA type is A3, A24, B8, B27, C2, C7, D2, D4.

A perfect match, when it comes to organ donation, will have all the same 8 HLA markers that you possess and display. In addition he or she must have the same red cell group of markers (those of the better know ABO system). Where can you find such a match? Outside the family circle your chances are poor indeed. That is why in the early days of transplantation a lot of 'living-related' organ transplantation was done. Naturally this was restricted to kidney transplantation for here we have a situation where there is one organ to spare, it is not too easy to talk family members into giving you a liver or a heart.

You do not have to be associated with a 'living donor' program for long before you become convinced that the immunological advantages are far outweighed by the disadvantages associated with the human drama involved.

To understand what I mean, put yourself through the following scenario. Your brother, five years your senior, is dying of kidney disease. Only a new kidney can save him; he is a kind, productive man with a dependent family. You are healthy and the only one in the family whose HLA type coincides with that of the sick man. Your brother hated to approach you to ask for such an incredible favour but, urged on by his wife and his parents, he put the question to you: 'Would you be willing to have a major operation to allow one of your two healthy kidneys to be removed so that it could replace my dead ones?'

All eyes are on you. What can you say? You are not happy about it, of course. It is a big operation. Things occasionally go wrong with surgery, don't they? You would be left with only one kidney and what if something happened to that, then you would be in a pretty fix! But you love your brother. The family want you to give him his chance. Things will never be the same if you say no and he died. A number of donors have told me that unavoidable pressures made it impossible for them to feel good about the selflessness of the act involved. They feel robbed of the satisfaction that comes with being quietly generous. Anyway, you go ahead with the operation and your brother has a new kidney. Imagine the feeling of all concerned if six weeks later the transplanted kidney is dead and the surgeons are back in again pulling out your now useless kidney. Your sacrifice has come to nothing.

Unfortunately, this can happen. While eighty to ninety per cent of so-called perfectly matched kidneys survive and indeed flourish, this is not always the case. The wound or the organ itself may become infected, the delicate hook up of the kidney to blood vessels and ureter (the tube that carries urine from the kidney to the bladder) may run into trouble or the recipient's immune system may reject the kidney after all.

His immune system can sometimes react to a slight difference that we could not pick up in our tissue typing program. This latter event needs a little explanation. There are undoubtedly 'trademark' antigens, of which we know little. With the exception of identical twins we cannot be one hundred per cent certain that two individuals, even family members, are perfectly matched. With families we can be 90 per cent sure and that is the state of the art. So it is that a sibling kidney may be rejected and the storms that burst when this sort of thing happens within a family are torrential. The donor is frustrated that his or her magnanimous gesture, with its anguish and discomfort, has failed. The recipient is overwhelmed by guilt at having rejected the sacrificed organ.

Because of the emotional tangle and because most patients with renal failure do not have a living relative who is a perfect match anyway, transplantation units have been forced to proceed with their work after accepting two compromises; they must harvest organs from the legally dead (cadaveric donors) and they must suppress the immune system of the new organ's recipient. Transplant teams try to get the best match possible for their patient but, in the real world, the immune system must be partially crippled for the transplanted organ to survive. The danger is easy to see. If you cannot reject the incompatible kidney you may not be able to reject the next virus that 'transplants' itself into your body.

What happens when a transplanted organ is attacked? It is a horrible thing to watch, I can tell you. The alarm sounding T cells recognise certain HLA proteins displayed on cells within the transplanted organ and its blood vessels. The alarm goes off and B and T cells swing into action, destroying the graft completely.

The immune system has a memory of elephantine proportions, as we know. Should a second transplant be attempted with tissue that resembles the first organ in any way, the graft can actually be rejected before the surgeon finishes stitching the new kidney into place. The kidney can swell up and turn black before the horrified eyes of the medical team.

There is nothing new under the sun and therefore nothing new about humanity's dream to replace old, worn or diseased parts with young healthy alternatives. There is a famous and very ancient painting of the saints Cosmos and Damian performing a transplant on a rich nobleman. A well-to-do man of stature needed a new leg and the donor, a black slave, is depicted in the painting in his now 'one-legged' state. There is a smile of intense satisfaction on his face at having been lucky enough to be asked to donate (after signing the appropriate informed consent sheet, of course), one of his legs. The black leg looks to be in good condition, attached to the thigh of the nobleman and there are absolutely no signs of the recipient being immunosuppressed. (Naturally, saints can control the immune system better than we can.)

The rest of us, however, must use powerful immunosuppressive drugs or paint to pull off such a trick. One of the big scandals of modern immunology involved a New York scientist working on ways to make white mice accept the transfer of skin from black mice. Pressures demanding success in the highly competitive world of academic medicine led him into a fatal trap for young players. He faked his success by painting a black square on the back of his white mice and hailing the 'hybrid' as a triumph for medical research. He was discovered and it checkmated his career.

Everyday, thousands of transplants are done as doctors and patients alike accept the compromises discussed above. A recent case can illustrate much that is involved. Eleven-year-old Carrie urgently needs a new liver. A year earlier, happy, average Carrie had the misfortune to be involved in a serious car accident. It was the last day of the Labor Day weekend and the family was racing up the New Jersey turnpike towards New York in heavy traffic and deteriorating weather conditions.

A car swerved recklessly into their lane; much too close for comfort. Carries' father braked, perhaps overreacting, and as a result the car spun, bounced, tumbled and stopped.

Both the parents and Carrie survived. Mother and father were wearing seat belts, Carrie was not. Her small body careened around the interior of the frenzied car, both bouncing and breaking apart. She awoke in an intensive care unit concussed, aching all over and reluctant to breathe as broken ribs protested. In the trauma her spleen, nestling under her left diaphragm, had ruptured and poured blood into her belly. Fortunately surgery had been in time to stop exsanguination but she had lost more than half of her blood volume.

None of this had any direct bearing on her need for a new liver. She could and did make a complete recovery from those dreadful injuries. What did Carrie more harm than the car accident, however, was the blood transfusion she was given to replace all the blood that she had lost as a result of the accident.

It was unbelievably bad luck that little Carrie was given a bottle of blood that was contaminated with a virus that can cause hepatitis (inflammation of the liver).

There are at least three hepatitis–producing viruses. Hepatitis A is a virus that enters our mouth, usually placed there by dirty fingers which pick the virus up from feces. It is often called 'infectious hepatitis', a silly name as all hepatitis is infectious. Hepatitis B is a disease one picks up either from blood or blood products or infected sexual secretions. It is spread in a manner that is identical to the spread of AIDS but it is far more infectious. Both hepatitis A and B can be screened for and all blood held in blood banks is checked to ensure that neither virus gets into a recipient. But a third hepatitis virus, perhaps even a fourth, fifth and sixth virus, spread very much like hepatitis B but currently cannot be detected in blood donated to the Red Cross or other similar sources. It is known as non −A non −B hepatitis. Usually it causes a mild transient inflammation of the liver and recovery follows. Not always, however. For Carrie the infection had flourished in her weakened state and destroyed too much of her liver for long-term survival to be possible.

Carrie was accepted by the liver transplant team and the hunt was on to find a liver. Carrie's cells were HLA typed and her profile fed into a computer. Any potential liver donor who, of course, would have to be involved in their own personal tragedy, would be screened so that the liver went to the best match waiting anywhere in the country.

No one thought there would be a chance of finding a perfect match, Carrie would be given one that was the best available but she would have to have her T and B cells blunted.

As expected, one person's tragedy was to be another's salvation. A call came from Tennessee. In an intensive care unit lay an eighteen-year-old girl shot in the head by her jealous boyfriend. Her brain was dead. The rest of her would soon follow. Distraught parents had given permission for organ harvesting. A team of surgeons from Carrie's hospital raced to an awaiting company jet, kindly and not uncommonly donated for the mission in hand. When they arrived three other teams would be waiting. One team from California wanted the girl's heart, another team wanted the kidneys and pancreas and another team would eventually get a chance to harvest the corneas of her eyes.

This sort of macabre but essential scavenging has become possible because of the widespread acceptance by the medical, legal, philosophical and theological communities that death of the brain is all that is needed to declare the death of a person. No longer must the heart stop beating and the chest stop rising before the harvesters can, with gratitude and appreciation of the sensitivities of all involved, extract life for the dying from the dead.

The liver was not too big for Carrie; fortunately the donor had been particularly small. In an eleven-hour operation Carrie's old liver was flung aside and the new organ placed into its new home. The surgeons triumphed and Carrie had a chance. Carrie was given a drug called cyclosporin, a sophisticated T cell poison. Unfortunately, it can be toxic to kidney and liver cells and must be used with the greatest of care. However, when administered with the appropriate skill, it can stop rejection with an acceptable degree of toxicity but the state of the transplantation art is still far from ideal.

What we need to do of course, is master the immunological manoeuvres that allow a pregnancy to survive. We must learn to make the immune system of an organ recipient accept a new organ as part of 'self' but continue to fight anything else that is foreign. Long-term immunosuppression is associated with high infection risks and an increased chance of developing cancer for reasons that will be explained later. Tolerance induction must be the way of the future.

In describing the immune system, you remember we discussed the remarkable fact that each and every lymphocyte is programmed to recognise one and only one specific antigen. If all those cells that can recognise a certain organ could be eliminated or paralysed, a graft could survive in an otherwise immunocompetent recipient. We can induce specific tolerance to an organ in a mouse or rat in this manner, but we cannot do it instantly. It takes days at least. With human transplantation, as soon as an organ is available it must be transplanted.

Research along a number of different lines seems promising. We are getting better and better at preserving organs in tissue culture conditions. If we could keep a kidney or liver alive and well for three to six weeks in an incubator before needing to transplant it, we could find the ultimate match for that organ, attempt to produce tolerance to that tissue in a prospective recipient and decrease the foreignness of the organ. It seems that with time in tissue culture, organs lose much of their HLA profile.

We know that T and B cells are at their most vulnerable to drugs when they divide. They must divide as part of their attack response to antigen. If we could develop drugs that would kill only those T cells and B cells dividing after an antigen challenge, we could eliminate all the cells capable of rejecting the organ. Such a mechanism is called clonal deletion (a clone is a family) and there is no doubt this will become a reality.

We can now activate special suppressor cells that will reduce the viciousness of aggressor cells that want to attack the liver or kidney or other transplanted tissue.

I want to return to the subject of bone marrow transplantation; important things are happening here that are revolutionising the treatment of one of the most lethal of diseases, leukemia. As usual we will illustrate the newer approaches by describing a case history.

Twenty-three-year-old Kay is a college student majoring in music. She is of Japanese American descent; looking Oriental and acting like an American. She presented herself to her campus medical office because she was unusually tired and weak. The pressure of examinations could not explain adequately her feelings, and especially the breathlessness that she was getting when walking up a flight of stairs. She was pale but otherwise looked well.

A routine blood count was performed and told the story. Kay had developed an acute form of leukemia. What does that mean? Leukemia is a cancerous expansion of white blood cells, i.e., an uncontrollable, unwanted and very dangerous proliferation. The chapter on cancer gives a much more detailed account of the drama that leads to cells misbehaving themselves so disastrously. It is important to understand that one of the hundreds of billions of T cells in Kay's body had become a renegade; only one cell is needed to develop this condition. The now cancerous cell divides incessantly and is soon crowding the spaces where T cells live and travel. Blood, lymph nodes, spleen and bone marrow fill up first, then the T cells spill out into the lungs and other tissues. In Kay's case they were also occupying part of her brain.

Now this is a real medical emergency. There was no time to worry about what treatment might do to normal cells and their infection-fighting capacity. If those malignant cells were not killed or at the very least hindered from their headlong rush to divide, there would be no Kay to worry about. Consequently, Kay was rushed into hospital and, that very day given intravenously five anti-cancer drugs known to be particularly effective against rapidly dividing cells. Normal cells in our bodies that must divide regularly will be damaged by these drugs. The cells most affected will be those that produce our hair, the cells lining the intestinal tract and, most dangerously, the normal cells in the bone marrow that produce for us platelets, red blood cells, B cells and the polymorphs and monocytes. All these cells are already in trouble anyway, because the leukemic cells are crowding them out, competing more than successfully for local nutrients.

Despite all this intensive treatment, Kay's malignant T cells continued to do their damage. We made the situation worse, not better, as we had not helped her cancer but damaged normal cells.

There are different forms of leukemia, depending on which of the leucocytes turns nasty. Monocytes and B cells can become leukemic. T cell leukemia is one of the worst forms of the disease and the results with Kay were unfortunately not unusual. The plan formulated to save Kay involved three risky 'ifs'. If we could find a suitable (not perfect) donor, we could try and kill *all* of Kay's cancer cells with doses of drugs and radiotherapy that would also kill *all* her normal marrow cells. We might have eliminated the cancer in this fashion but to survive Kay needed a transplant of normal cells that would once again supply her with the essential elements of blood. If a perfect donor could not be found, one as close as possible was necessary to minimise the risks involved in this sort of procedure. Help was needed from the computer. We would also use new techniques to take from the donated bone marrow as many T cells as possible. If we could get rid of every last cell there would be no danger from graft versus host disease. The fastidiousness with which we approach this T cell elimination is terribly important as animal experiments have shown that it can take but one T cell to kill a helplessly immunodeficient mouse.

Kay was lucky with the computer; a man in England was willing to travel to America to give her his almost identical marrow. Five of the eight major antigens matched and Kay was prepared for her 'one chance' ordeal. Her body was treated with massive doses of anti-cancer drugs and she was irradiated. She was nursed in a specialised sterile room, equipped with sophisticated air conditioning that ensured that air that went out did not return, while air that did come into the room was treated with ultraviolet light. Everyone entering the room was as clean as was practicable. Doctors and nurses showered and entered the room masked, gloved and gowned. The donor arrived, met Kay and her family, (the heartwarming part of this sort of adventure), was anesthetised and the donation proceeded. One hundred and forty-two times the surgeons inserted needles deep into the bones of his hip to aspirate from the depths those precious marrow cells needed.

Once obtained, the cells were rushed to a sterile laboratory where an attempt was made to remove all the donor's T cells. For some reason, T cells have a characteristic that makes them stick to sheep (and only sheep) red blood cells. We added some sterile sheep red blood cells to the marrow and many of the T cells present clumped together with the red cells. We then spun the whole preparation in a centrifuge and a large number of the T cells in the preparation fell to the bottom of our tubes because they were heavy now that they were attached to the red blood cells. Carefully we aspirated the top layer and then added some extracts from peanuts which, of all things, are known to clump T cells. We spun the preparation again. For twelve hours we repeated these steps over and over again until less than one in a hundred of the cells left in the marrow appeared to be T cells. It was not perfect but it was the best we could do.

The T-depleted cells were transfused into Kay. We gave her more drugs to cover the possibility that a few T cells in the marrow donated might have been ready to attack her. We gave her large amounts of antibodies obtained from normal blood. We kept everything sterile and waited. (It takes a month before we can judge success or failure.) Kay needed infusions of normal people's platelets and polymorphs. She needed lots of sophisticated antibiotics. The blood transfusions we gave her were first irradiated to make sure that no live T cells were present in the transfusion.

Kay's graft took and she was well. The leukemia may still return, however. Of course, we hope it will not but if we left alive even a few leukemic cells at the time we were preparing her for the transplant then the disease would recur. However, she had her chance; something she would not have had with the same condition even a few years ago.

Kay's operation and general expenses cost about $100,000. The job is technically demanding and very labor-intensive, needing a great number of doctors and nurses with special skills. We must hope that our ability to manipulate the defensive system of man will soon allow us to handle these conditions with far less danger and expense.

It may surprise you to learn that of all the transplantation procedures, heart transplantation is the easiest and most successful. This was not always so, but there have been remarkable advances in this work. Transplanting hearts and lungs simultaneously, which unfortunately we often need to do, remains less satisfactory though is improving all the time. Kidneys, liver, skin, bone marrow, hearts and eye tissue are regularly and successfully transplanted. Pancreatic transplantation (which theoretically could cure diabetes) is not as yet successful, but the research into this form of therapy is proceeding well. Nervous tissue (nerves and the brain itself) remain notoriously difficult to transplant and are likely to remain so. It is not the immunology that is so difficult here but the problem of connections. Imagine a table filled with spaghetti. A sharp knife divides all of the segments into two. The two halves are then separated and presented to you with instructions to join up all the pieces so that the original configuration is renewed. Such a task would be easy when compared to joining up the many millions of elements that make up our nervous tissue.

While we have emphasised many of the problems associated with transplantation, we must remember that transplantation today is saving many lives. In Sydney recently a wedding was held that was more than a little unusual. Both the bride and groom had undergone a heart transplant operation successfully. After they were declared man and wife and embraced each other and their parents, they turned to embrace the parents of the two young people whose hearts beat inside them. I am sure the loss of the two people who had donated those hearts was made more bearable at that moment.

PART III THE DEFEAT OF THE WARRIORS

5 | The topic of cancer

W HAT is so intrinsically disturbing about cancer? Everyone knows it is a process that can kill, and so we humans, constantly if subconsciously concerned about the brevity of life, are naturally fightened of something that is so often responsible for our demise.

One in four of you reading this book will die of cancer. But is the knowledge that a tumor may kill us a good enough explanation for the dread that is conjured by the term 'cancer'? After all, more of us will die of heart problems than of cancer, yet the thought of a heart attack, although distressing, is more tolerable than the thought of cancer.

Perhaps in that sentence I have stumbled upon the reason why cancer is so feared. We know we can survive heart attack, we may indeed live with it, but cancer? How many people do we know who have been cured of cancer? In fact, many people are cured of some forms of cancer, but little publicity is given to such advances.

I doubt, however, that the perception that death will certainly follow the development of cancer is responsible for its reputation as the most feared of diagnoses. As is so often the case with physicians, my understanding of people's attitudes towards cancer was considerably broadened by one of my patients.

Jennifer was an excellent nurse who had worked in our outpatient department for many years. Forty-nine years old, the mother of four, and the caregiver to an aged mother, she had always been healthy apart from some chronic but not debilitating bronchitis. One day, however, she confided to me that she was concerned because she had coughed up some blood three mornings in a row. There was little else to tell; she had no pain, no deterioration in well being although she admitted to having lost some weight in recent months. I arranged for her to have an X-ray examination of her chest. Already advanced cancer, starting in the bronchial tree and progressing to eat its way into her lungs, stood out in bold relief from the normal structures of the chest so clearly displayed on the picture obtained.

Of course, it is harder to deliver bad news to a colleague than it is to a stranger and I am sure you will understand that such episodes are emotionally charged. After we had discussed the matter for some minutes Jennifer asked whether she could see the X-ray film, not doubting the information, of course, but instantly summoning the defiance that humans can harness to defend their psyche. She stared at the film for a long time after I had explained that it would not be possible to eradicate the growth surgically. The silence was heavy. Eventually after what seemed like minutes, she turned to me.

'It's not the picture on the screen that is so devastating to me,' she said quietly. 'It is what lies ahead for me and my family. That's what I see when I look at that X-ray. I know what dying from cancer will entail.'

From this and similar conversations, I believe it is the connotation of a protracted battle with a high chance of defeat that frequently colours the diagnosis of cancer with great, indeed unwarranted fear.

Cancer is a doubly frustrating condition for the clinical scientist. Failure to help patients in their struggle with cancer has, until recently, been shared with the failure to understand the grossly disordered biological processes responsible for this suffering; all this at a time when other complex medical problems are being rapidly solved. Fortunately, all that is changing rapidly and thus the tone of this chapter can definitely be one of optimism.

At this point, you may be wondering why cancer is being discussed in a book about the immune system. The answer is simple. Certain cancerous cells can, albeit with difficulty, be distinguished from normal cells. We have every reason to believe that lymphocytes can recognise these differences. We also know that lymphocytes can and frequently do kill certain tumor cells. The questions therefore that immunologists must face are these: is clinically advanced cancer the result of a failure of our immune systems? Are our immune systems charged with the responsibility of constantly screening self to detect cancerous changes in bone, breast or bowel, etc.? If so, is cancer an immunodeficiency disease? Should all cancer cells be recognised as dangerous by our immune system, or are some clever enough to be indistinguishable from self and thus capable of tricking the most perfect of immune systems?

These are the concepts that we must explore. Understanding the answers to these questions would provide not only a breakthrough in our knowledge of cancerous growth but new and logical ways to approach the treatment of malignancy.

To be logical, we must first explore those events that transform a once normal cell into a renegade, disobeying all the regulatory signals it has hitherto obeyed. Once we understand why the cell has so drastically changed its character and function, we can explore its interaction, or lack thereof, with the immune system.

Jennifer developed cancer in a fraction of a second. At one moment she did not have cancer, at the next moment she did. In that split second, the normal functioning of one cell was permanently disarrayed. In that moment, perhaps months or even years before clinical disease developed, her fate was settled. In her case one cell somewhere among the billions of similar cells that lined her airways (bronchial tree) took the malignant approach to its future biological role.

It divided and divided, producing an ever expanding family of identical cells with identical attitudes towards control. With abandon these cells spread and invaded, damaging normal tissues as they ruthlessly pursued their quest for immortality. At the most fundamental level, that is what cancer is all about — immortality. Only the failure of the cancer victim to sustain the nutritional requirements of the cancerous cell's growth frustrates these tumors' intention.

Increasingly, scientists are able to put single cancer cells in a test tube inside an incubator and observe their apparent immortality. As long as they are fed they live, they multiply. Not so normal cells; their mortality in such artificial systems is obvious within days.

We understand that normal cells in any part of the body have, as an integral part of their genetic makeup, clearly laid out instructions for growth and differentiation (development of a specific function) and division (replication of self). Each and every normal cell is under the tightest of control mechanisms. The cell is programmed from its conception to its death; very definitely, the latter is preprogrammed into the cell. It will divide a finite number of times, then it will die. The simultaneous death of a critical mass of cells in a vital organ will lead to our death. As we age, cells that have the capacity to repair tissues and even repair damaged genetic material die. We are welcome guests of our biological environment, but only for so long.

On the other hand, cancer cells have broken loose from the shackles of self-imposed mortality. They have turned off the biological timer inside their nucleus that would tell them when to self-destruct. The irony is all too obvious; in achieving their chance for immortality, they accelerate the death of normal cells that surround them and ultimately in so doing they destroy themselves. We now know that as we humans age, cells rebel and become cancerous much more easily. We also know that every cell in our body has the potential for malignant change.

Cancer is thus a disease process in which one cell undergoes an internal rearrangement of its instructive material so that it no longer lives by the laws of ordered biological development and demise. It stimulates its own growth and replication. It loses its biological death wish and necessarily invades and spreads into both adjoining and remote corners of the body as it reproduces itself endlessly, and in so doing produces damaging mass effects.

How does such a disastrous turn of events occur? Two factors must be considered together. First, we will explore the concept that all cells have the potential to become malignant, then we will look at what is known of triggering factors that may impact upon a cell and unleash its tendency to indulge in malignant behaviour.

Look at the back of your hand. Does it look the same to you as it did a month ago? It probably does, but it isn't. Many of the cells you see there, neatly glued together to make skin, were not present a month ago. Much of our body is continuously dying and being replaced in a vital process imperceptible to us in our day-to-day life.

This need to shed and repair puts us at increased risk of developing cancer. Normal cells are turned on and told to divide and, having done so, are then very definitely turned off. The complexities involved in this signalling put us at risk should the system falter and the turnoff signals be ignored.

However, before discussing, these things, we shall return to the story of the nurse Jennifer. To confirm a diagnosis and determine the type of cancer in her lungs, a tube was manoeuvred down her throat and trachea into her bronchial tree. Using warm saline, her airways were lavaged, and the cells washed out from deep in her chest were examined under the microscope. Their malignant nature was readily identified. After consultation with radiotherapists, surgeons and physicians skilled in the poisoning by chemicals of tumor cells, it was decided that radiation therapy offered the best chance of slowing the spread of her disease. Bravely, Jennifer commenced her battle against cancer. The scenario she had anticipated became reality with unerring accuracy, until one remarkable departure from the normal script occurred.

Her cancer was mainly confined to the upper portion of her right lung. Eventually in its outward push it reached that part of the lung closest to the chest wall. The lung there is lined by a thin filmy layer called the pleura. (Sometimes it becomes infected and when you take a deep breath it stretches and hurts; that is called pleurisy.) The inside of your ribcage is lined by pleura also, and the layer over the lung and that on your chest wall move easily over each other when we breathe. An oily liquid lubricates their surface, so normally these movements are frictionless.

Jennifer's cancer, which had started from her airways, burst from her lung into this pleural space. Now when she tried to breathe, air would

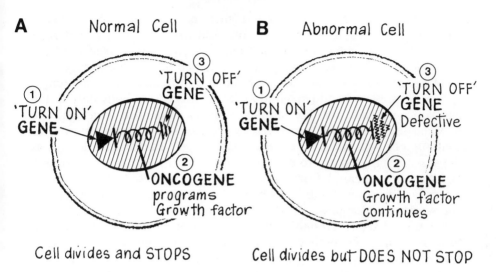

A Normal Cell

① 'TURN ON' GENE

③ 'TURN OFF' GENE

② ONCOGENE programs Growth factor

Cell divides and STOPS

B Abnormal Cell

① 'TURN ON' GENE

③ 'TURN OFF' GENE Defective

② ONCOGENE Growth factor continues

Cell divides but DOES NOT STOP

A VIRUS carrying ONCOGENE

moves into NUCLEUS

CANCER

B Cell now dividing out of control

INFECTIOUS VIRUS CARRYING ONCOGENE secretion of many new viral parts carrying oncogenes move along the cancerous track into that space, which filled up like a balloon expanding. The pressures collapsed the other part of her right lung and, as you would expect, she felt pain and breathlessness. Worse was to follow. Bacteria from her airways settled in her pleural space and an abscess formed at that site. It extended into the cancer-ridden lung.

Jennifer shivered and perspired as fevers racked her body despite the antibiotics we gave her. For ten days she was suspended on a tightrope between life and death. Jennifer however, was tough and survived to continue her fight with cancer. But what cancer? Remarkable to tell, as the abscess settled down to be replaced by scar tissue, her tumor shrank and then disappeared from view. Three years later as I write these words, and two and a half years beyond her date with death, she is well and working and appears to be free of tumor.

A miracle? Well, certainly miraculous in the sense of being an unusual turn of events, but perhaps the miracle was wrought by her immune system. Lymphocytes might well have been the minions of the Almighty in saving this worthy lady in a most unusual fashion. An extremely important consideration concerns the delineation of the mechanisms that could have cured this nurse. We will return to this subject later.

Before we continue our discussion of the inner working of cells, we should define a few terms to ensure that what follows is readily understandable. The study of the heart in health and disease is called cardiology; the study of the cell that has become cancerous is called oncology ('onco' from the Greek *onkos* meaning 'mass' or 'tumor'). A doctor who specialises in cancer is an oncologist.

The concept of malignancy is not a medical one alone; malignant is the opposite of benign. Both terms are used frequently when describing swellings (tumors) found in the body. Not all tumors are cancerous expansions, for they can be benign and therefore of little concern.

All of which brings us back to the most important discovery in the field of cancer research in the past twenty years — oncogenes; genes that can cause cancer.

In 1910 in New York city a young scientist, Dr Francis Rous was studying cancer in animals at the famous Rockefeller Institute for Medical Research. His work received some publicity and as a result a most important meeting occurred. An astute farmer was troubled because some of his Plymouth Rock hens were developing tumors that would eventually kill them. The farmer decided he would consult the bright young Dr Rous about his observations and took one of his affected hens to the Institute. Rous was fascinated because these 'cancers' seemed to be infectious; too many of the farmer's hens were infected for the cancer to be random.

Rous got to work and was soon able to show that if a small piece of the tumor was taken and implanted in another hen of the same strain, similar cancers developed. In a series of now quite famous experiments, Rous was able to show that the cancer-initiating substance was smaller than a cell, smaller in fact than bacteria, for he could still produce cancers after passing the tumor tissue through the smallest of the then available filters. Rous postulated that cancer might be caused by a virus.

What we are talking about is in no way similar to the manner in which viruses may cause the common cold. In that situation viruses take up residence in say, the nose, multiply and get themselves attacked by the immune system, which wins, but not without a lot of suffering. Your nose becomes the battlefield for the biological war.

In the cancer context we are inferring that viruses, which are nothing but collections of genetic information, insinuate themselves into cells and change their programming system in such a way that they proliferate in the manner described earlier. A number of viruses can do this and many have been discovered and studied in the animal world. Those studied most thoroughly are, interestingly enough, viruses that belong to the same family to which belongs the virus that causes AIDS.

How do viruses turn a respectable well-behaved cell into a killer? This is where the oncogenes come in. Certain viruses include in their genetic repertoire genes that are capable of stimulating malignant growth in invaded (parasitised) cells. These will be interwoven with the genetic information that the victimised cell will need if it is to do its new master's will and produce more virus.

But why would a virus wish to turn its host cell into a cancer cell? Cancer cells constantly divide and it is during division that viruses most effectively reproduce. Needless to say, the virus cares not for the fate of the invaded cell.

There is still a missing link to be discussed that bridges the gap between the virus and the cancerous behaviour. Genes, as we have discussed, instruct cells to make a specific product. They supply blueprints for the formation of specific proteins, that is, chemicals that influence biological function. The inference here therefore is that proteins, produced by an infected cell, in response to the message delivered by oncogenes, can actually *cause* cancerous growth. The virus Rous discovered can certainly do just that.

Having discussed this, we must immediately point out that there is a major problem with this scenario (viral oncogenes triggering cancer) as an explanation for all malignant growth. Most cancers, especially in humans, cannot be related to viral infection at all. This puzzle only started to take better shape with the recent and most significant discovery that oncogenes can be found in normal human cells not infected with viruses.

This sensational discovery has ruined a number of hitherto prestigious hypotheses. Oncogenes in normal cells! Has nature gone mad? Millions of animals, both human and otherwise die each year from cancers occurring in so many tissues. Surely such a fundamental design flaw should have been rooted out of our biological systems by this stage of the evolutionary process.

A more calculating and less emotional look at Nature's priorities partially answers the question: we must not live forever if the species is to survive. In the case of us humans, Nature could hardly be expected to have anticipated that so many of us would be sedentary, obese and hooked on cholesterol and alcohol and therefore depart ahead of time from heart attacks and other diseases. Cancer could be seen as Nature's final solution to the hazard that is longevity. We know, for example, that if men live long enough they all develop cancer in their prostate glands. Thus we have oncogenes occasionally being delivered by viruses but other cells seem to be able to get into trouble by producing their own oncogenes.

The oncogene story, however, is even more fascinating than this scenario would suggest. These genes are present in normal cells and many if not all of them are owned by the cell. They are not bad genes dumped there by a passing virus. In a fascinating turn around, it seems that oncogenes actually 'infect' viruses. Here is how these mechanisms could produce cancer by infection.

Meet Richard, a tired, middle-order executive who, as we are introduced, is hanging on to the support strap as a suburban train jerks him home from work. His day at the office was a bad one, and he is looking forward to a cold beer with his wife, to whom he can pour out the frustrations of the day. A multitude of thoughts race through his mind, but he is not thinking about the cell at the back of his throat that has become malignant. In two months, it will result in a small tumor that will touch his vocal cords. In six months he will first notice a little hoarseness. In twelve months he will be subjected to necessarily mutilating surgery and will have no voicebox at all. Here's hoping he survives. But all that is in the future; a more immediate biological drama is about to unfold.

Enter character No 2 in this theatre of life. Samuel is swaying as the train lurches. He is hanging on to a strap three away from the one clutched by Richard. Samuel is back at work today for the first time in a week as he has been recovering from an upper respiratory tract infection. In the crowded train carriage Samuel, to his embarrassment, is taken over by the irresistible urge to sneeze. He tries to shield his nose but an explosive sneeze occurs; not a soul seems to notice.

With that sneeze six million viral particles are released into the air. Some will settle on the floor, others on clothes and newspapers, some will be swirling in the air that Richard quietly inhales as he waits for his journey to end.

One of those viral particles lands on the surface of the cancerous cell at the back of Richard's throat. It burrows through the cell membrane and makes for the cell's nucleus. Here is a haven in which it will temporarily settle while it makes more of itself. Soon the cell is making more viral particles that will eventually burst out of the cell, ready to infect other cells locally or be coughed out into the environment, looking for a fresh host.

In the particular cell that has become home to Samuel's virus, there is already a problem. The cell's oncogenes have activated a growth pattern that is cancerous. As the cell makes viral particles (which are in fact, viral genes) they can pick up an activated oncogene, hard at work in this cancerous cell. That is, the new viral particles being produced have added an activated oncogene to their genetic makeup and this they will take with them to the next cell they infect. When they infect that cell with their passenger oncogene, they could initiate a malignant change in that cell. In such a manner, cancer can be 'infectious'. Next time Richard coughs in the train he will expose others not only to Samuel's virus but to activated oncogenes as well.

This turns out to be the fuller explanation of the cancer in hens studied by Dr Rous all those years ago. The virus he found did not cause the cancer; it just carried the cancer-activating signal from one hen to the next. Virally induced cancer can thus follow infection with a virus that possesses its own oncogene, or simply carries a cancer-promoting gene, 'donated' by a previously infected cell. There is no doubt that this viral-mediated threat is an important one, but it is not the major way that cancers develop.

To examine the next step in the unravelling of the cause of cancer, we need to return to the apparent enigma presented to us with the discovery that normal cells possess oncogenes. At first scientists regarded these oncogenes as time-bombs: the genes would sit in the cell in a quiescent fashion until either some intrinsic biological timer said 'fire' or the cell was disturbed by a process that would prematurely trigger the explosion that would lead to cancer. In this view of the cellular drama, oncogenes can only be looked upon as genes that Nature has designed for destructive purposes. New information, however, puts the oncogene problem into better perspective.

Oncogenes are not intrinsically bad genes. They do not sit in cells with nothing to do but wait for the day when they will initiate a tragedy. The truth is that they are constantly playing a role in the most important activity of any cell: self-replication.

Alcohol is not evil, but we all know how 'malignant' can be the effects of uncontrolled overindulgence in this drug. 'Control', 'discipline' and 'appropriate' are all words that conjure up the connotations associated with the harmless consumption of alcohol. And so it is with oncogenes. When they are controlled all is well; when they are not, cancer results.

To understand this part of the story we must ask what is known about the 'normal' function of oncogenes. All the genes, as we have said repeatedly, instruct cells to produce proteins that have a biological function. The proteins produced by oncogenes are vital for replication and therefore the growth or repair of our tissues.

In 1975 a well known scientist interested in cell replication summed up this aspect of cellular life in this way: 'the most extraordinary attribute of living organisms is their capacity for precise self-replication, a property that can be regarded as a very quintessence of the living estate.'

Professor Lehningen was not talking about the propagation of a species. When a man and a woman produce a baby, that is not self-replication; rather it is the creation of unique newness. We are discussing the replication of self—the replacement-of-skin-on-the-back-of-the-hand concept discussed earlier. It turns out that oncogenes are essential for the orderly process of cell division necessary for a cell to reproduce itself. Such a process is known as mitosis. Only when something goes wrong with oncogene performance does cancer develop. For this reason oncogenes were, in reality, badly named and of course, have had a lot of bad press as biological villains. They should have been called mitogenes.

So, we can put the cancer story into perspective. A cell is only one tiny component of a mighty system. Genes constantly issue instructions to the cell to produce something vital to the mass effort of the organ (move that leg, pump that blood, produce that insulin, etc.). At a precisely *ordered* moment in the cell's hectic life, regulator genes activate oncogenes and suppress other instructions. The oncogenes swing into action and the cellular mechanisms involved in one becoming two proceeds apace.

With divisions safely accomplished, oncogenes are switched off by another set of regulatory genes, often located next to the oncogenes on a certain chromosome. If an activated oncogene is divorced from its control mechanisms (picked up by a virus, for example) or if its control mechanisms are disturbed, orderly division is lost and cells are told to continually replicate. They divide and divide again. As they continue in this fashion, a tumor (mass) is formed and a cancerous growth with all its inherent hazards is born.

A most important question for cancer scientists can therefore be posed. What are the factors that can activate oncogenes, disturb their regulation and thus promote the development of cancer? Much progress is being made in this vital area. It is certain that external factors are not always necessary for the disordered regulation of cell division to occur; things can and do go wrong inside the cell with no help from the outside world. But many, perhaps most, cancers involve derangement of oncogene control by environmental factors, e.g., asbestos in the lungs can cause lung cancer.

We have already discussed viruses in some detail but even better studied are cancer-promoting chemicals; the so-called carcinogens. Numerous chemicals can interfere with the DNA message possessed by the oncogene and its controlling forces.

In rats the administration of nitrosomethylurea causes breast cancer by changing the DNA message very subtly. The effects are anything but subtle, however; oncogenes are activated in breast cells and cancer develops.

We live in a 'chemical world', all of us are constantly exposed to naturally occurring and synthesised chemicals, be they in the form of preservatives in food, drugs from the pharmacist's shelf or additives to gasoline. The wonder is that of all the chemicals to which we are exposed, relatively few have carcinogenic potential. It follows, then, that most cancer in humans is triggered by other factors, or occurs spontaneously. That in no way should diminish our determination to find and eliminate from our environment those elements that do have the potential for causing cancer.

The discussion of cancer is now at the point where we must stop and examine the question of cigarette smoking. The tar, chemicals and nicotine contained in cigarettes are far and away the most dangerous chemical carcinogens in our environment, and to do anything but explore this issue thoroughly would not be appropriate. I will try and do this unemotionally, but it is not easy. Physicians see so much unnecessary suffering directly resulting from smoking that it is hard to be dispassionate about the subject, given our miserable track record in getting people to stop the habit and, even more importantly, to refrain from starting.

You remember Jennifer, of course; lucky Jennifer, as it turns out. Well, she was seldom seen socially without a cigarette between her lips. Her bronchitis was caused by smoking more than thirty cigarettes a day for more than thirty years. The simple inescapable fact is that smoking kills and kills and kills. That tobacco manufacturers should be allowed to glamorise this deadly product is a disgrace in an informed society. Tobacco companies employ smooth, verbally skilled individuals to constantly pour doubt on the scientific community's protestations, which are based on ever more convincing evidence, that cigarette smoking is a health hazard of major proportions. It is very different from the situation with alcohol.

Studies support the concept that moderate alcohol intake is harmless. No degree of smoking is harmless; even one low-tar cigarette a week poses risks that should be seen as unacceptable. In fact as we will discuss, inhaling someone else's smoke (i.e., passive smoking) is also dangerous.

Why is smoking so dangerous? Ignoring for the moment all the non-malignant hazards of smoking, the fact is that the chemicals associated with tar, combined with the blood-vessel-changing properties of nicotine, irritate cells to such an extent that deregulation of oncogene activity is a predictable outcome. If you sniff tobacco into your nose you can get cancer in your nose. If you chew tobacco or smoke a pipe, you are at great risk of developing cancer in your mouth. If you inhale it into your airways, the cells lining your bronchial tree are poisoned day in and day out. Hundreds and thousands of Jennifers find out about tar and oncogenes in the most devastating fashion each year.

Cigarette smoking causes bronchitis that may lead to destruction of lung tissue (emphysema). It promotes the development of stomach ulcers and clots in veins. The latter can break away from walls of veins and race to the lungs or brain, causing terrible damage. Cigarettes promote the development of varicose veins, dangerously lower the birth weight of babies if mothers smoke during pregnancy and very markedly increase the risk of developing heart disease. Smokers, on average, have 30 per cent more sick days per year than do individuals who do not smoke. The combination of oral contraceptives and smoking increases the risk of a woman over thirty-five having a heart attack thirty-nine times and the risk of having a stroke twenty-two times. Women who are heavy smokers run a much greater risk of developing cancer of the cervix. Smoking lowers fertility in both males and females.

In most Western countries, smoking is responsible for five times more deaths per year than traffic accidents. In the United States of America, where men can expect to live beyond seventy years of age, forty per cent of smokers who use twenty-five or more cigarettes per day die before the age of forty-five. Habitual twenty-per-day smokers shorten their life span, on average, by at least five years; many reduce it much more than that.

If you like playing games with statistics you can calculate that the average smoker shortens his life by 5.5 minutes with each cigarette he or she smokes. Men below the age of forty-five who smoke fifteen cigarettes per day or more are nine times more likely to die of coronary heart disease than men of the same age who do not smoke.

The figures are overwhelming, the scientific facts indisputable. Yet the percentage of individuals who smoke, especially women, is increasing in most countries. Governments can be roundly criticised for their capitulation to the rich tobacco industry. All forms of cigarette advertising should be banned and warnings on packages should scream 'smoking kills'.

Physicians, educators, sociologists and psychologists have totally failed to develop strategies that will significantly reduce the incidence of young people taking up smoking. What twelve-year-old cares what his health will be like when he is forty? Perhaps the only hope for the near future is the increasingly common attitude among non-smokers that smoking is indeed an antisocial habit. Expense, bad breath, ash litter, etc., have never deterred smokers but if smoking is regarded by society as an antisocial, disgusting, foolish, non-macho weakness, then we may get somewhere.

The rapidly accumulating evidence that inhaling someone else's smoke (passive smoking) is dangerous may just turn the tide. Sociological change, not medical facts, influence societal smoking patterns. Restaurants, aircraft, and the workplace are just some of the commonly encountered spaces in which those who do not care to smoke are affected by the smoke produced by others in the area.

Smoke is an interesting and dangerous substance. Watch a puff of smoke from some smoker's mouth and you will see that the smoke flows can be divided into mainstream and sidestream sections. The latter is likely to drift into your area and therefore be taken into your lungs. Because of its dispersion properties, sidestream smoke contains considerably more of the most dangerous chemicals than does mainstream smoke. For example, in sidestream smoke there is more carbon monoxide, tar and nicotine than is found in mainstream smoke. Three-quarters of the nicotine retained by filter tip cigarettes is released into the air in sidestream smoke. As a result the majority of non-smokers have nicotine detectable in their body fluids most of their lives. It has been calculated that an office worker sharing space with a smoker may inhale the equivalent of five cigarettes per day.

One can go on and on, and certainly the most polite and timid among us must deliver an emphatic 'yes' to the question, 'Do you mind if I smoke?' But we are talking about cancer and it is no exaggeration to say that lung cancer would be reduced by more than ninety-five per cent if people did not smoke. Not that lung cancer is the only malignancy associated with smoking, as we have discussed.

Given the expense, the suffering and the death caused by smoking, we all have a responsibility to remain educated about this matter and to do our part in removing this definite cause of cancer and so many other ills.

Many other environmental factors interact with cells to trigger cancerous changes. Overcooked food can cause bowel cancer (Japanese communities in which only raw fish is consumed have no cancer of the intestinal tract); expatriate Japanese from such areas living in other sites where they eat cooked food have the same chance of getting cancer as do the locals. The hepatitis B virus can precipitate the development of cancer of the liver. The virus that causes glandular fever (infectious mononucleosis) can cause cancer in the throat and cancer in B lymphocytes. Hundreds of other examples could be given.

To summarise, cancer occurs when the process of orderly self-replication is disturbed. Oncogenes are activated either spontaneously (intrinsically) or by chemicals, viruses or other extrinsic factors. If these activated genes are not rapidly deactivated, cell division will continue in an uncontrolled fashion; a tumor will develop. This mass of cells will crush local, normal tissue and the cells will break down walls of blood and lymphatic vessels. Cancer cells will then be transplanted (metastatised) to different parts of the body, there to continue their deadly expansion. Vital organs will be damaged and the patient will die.

At last, then, we come to the immunology of cancer. Let's set the scene. A cell has, for one reason or another, embarked upon a malignant course. Is the cell still self or is it foreign? This question has been challenging the scientific community for fifty years or more, as the answer is of utmost importance. If cancer cells are self, albeit dangerous, then there is no reason for lymphocytes to attack and destroy them. If they are, in their malignant state, even slightly different from self, then they should be killed. Cancer could then be at least partially blamed on an inefficient immune system.

Fifty years ago scientists took tumors from animals and implanted them into other animals. The recipients' immune systems mounted a vicious attack and soon disposed of the unwanted tumor cells. The researchers claimed, not unreasonably, that cancer cells could be rejected by immune mechanisms and inferred that the donor's immune system was defective. The problem was that the animals rejected the cancer, not because it was cancer, but because it was foreign tissue. Transplant rejection rather than cancer rejection was being observed.

While this situation was being sorted out, clinicians had no doubts about the matter. Patients who are immunosuppressed, either by disease or treatment, have a significantly increased risk of developing cancer. Nowhere is this more obvious than in patients who have undergone an organ transplantation. A patient harboring someone else's kidney needed that new kidney for survival; his immune system cannot be allowed to reject the donated tissue. When drugs are used to blunt our immune response to the organ transplanted, the incidence of cancer developing in the patient is increased. Obviously some homeostatic mechanism has been compromised.

From such observations came two related ideas. The first idea suggests that cancer cells must be developing fairly frequently in everyone's body, while the second suggests that the normal but potentially dangerous situation is controlled by competent lymphocytes that recognise a cell's malignant change and then destroy it. All day, every day, lymphocytes carry out 'immunological surveillance' to ensure the early detection of cancer. Both ideas have been confirmed as fact.

With the development of our ability to 'stage' an attack by the immune system on cancer cells in a test tube, we have been able to demonstrate that at least three distinct cell types within the immune system can kill tumor cells. A branch of the T cell family 'cytotoxic' T cells, can attack tumor cells physically, grappling with their membranes and then destroying them.

A second group of cancer-killing cells are called natural killer cells. These are lymphocyte lookalikes, dependent on the availability of interferon to activate their chemical attack on tumor cells. Finally there are K cells, a lymphocyte-like cell that can kill (hence the capital K) tumor cells coated with antibody to some component of the cancer cell wall. The antibody guides the K cell to the target.

To kill a cancer cell, the cell, metaphorically speaking, has to stick its tongue out at the potential killer cells; there must be something on the surface of the cancer cell that declares its renegade state. In addition, you may remember, T cells at least can only attack when simultaneously they see 'self' in the form of histocompatibility antigens at the same time as they see foreignness. Thus we can only expect killing of cancer cells if they display 'tumor-specific antigens' and a self moiety *simultaneously* on their cell membranes.

Fortunately for us, most of the time they do just this and they are killed. There is a 'new you' coming every day, all right, eight billion cells you did not have yesterday, some of which are malignant. Day in day out, we kill off new but cancerous cells before they can do any harm.

The problem is that, in certain tissues, tumors may arise that display precious few of these essential 'give away' markers. What's more, they may protect themselves in at least two ways. Firstly, they may deliberately hide those telltale cancer markers on their surface and secondly, they may activate regulatory T cells in the environment around them to blunt the attack against themselves. Pretty clever, you will agree.

There is a familial component in all this cancer immunology. As with so much of biological performance, some of us are better at handling cancer than are others. This variable degree of proficiency may apply to cancer in general or perhaps just to cancer occurring in certain tissues.

Here is a true case history to illustrate this. Margaret noted a small lump in her right breast when she was thirty-six years old. It was removed surgically and found to be a cancer. Caught early enough, all cancers that can be removed can be cured. While you never can be certain, however, that a few cells have not escaped, Margaret was still well five years later and so considered one of the lucky ones.

At forty-seven years of age, a routine smear from the mouth of her womb showed an early stage of cancer. Again the surgeon removed malignant tissue to save her. At fifty-one, she was enjoying good health, as she had been since that operation. Recently, however, she had noticed some blood in her stool. Not visible blood, but blood that she could detect by using a chemically impregnated card that reacts to it.

Why was Margaret so compulsive in seeking blood in her stool?

Margaret's mother had died at the age of fifty-two from cancer of the colon. Her two aunts had also died of cancer before their sixtieth birthdays. One had a tumor in the pancreas and the other cancer in her colon. Margaret's grandmother had died of cancer starting somewhere in her genital tract. Margaret's sister had breast cancer and had not been as lucky as Margaret; she was alive but the tumor was in her liver.

Cancers plague some families in a manner such as this, and while not particularly common, it occurs frequently enough for us to realise that genetically inherited influences can predispose generations to cancer. As blood in the stool is often a very early sign of cancer of the bowel, Margaret had been advised to check her stool in the way described. With the detection of the blood a colonoscopy (examination of the colon with a flexible tube that features fiber optics to allow one to look around corners) was performed. An early cancer was found and removed by the instruments attached to the colonscope. Margaret battles on.

There is evidence to suggest that the propensity to cancer development, shown by Margaret's family, may also be inherited by individuals rather than families.

We have already said that, the second time an antigen is encountered, the stronger will be the body's immune response to that particular substance. Once sensitised, immunological memory supplies a much higher level of protection. If cells are taken from a tumor and put in a test tube, then T cells are taken from the blood of a healthy person picked at random, not much happens immediately. The T cells are not sensitised to the cancer. They have never seen such tissue before.

But with certain tumors, if T cells are taken not from the proverbial 'man in the street' but from a healthy but close physical associate of the patient with cancer, not necessarily a family member, things may be quite different. The T cells of lovers, flatmates, family members living in the same house, or other close associates, often rapidly attack the tumor cells obtained from their close contact. One conclusion seems inescapable; all these people with sensitised T cells have met and defeated the same cancer in their own bodies or they have 'seen' and become immune to the cancer-triggering chemical or other cause that is now displayed on the surface of their friend's tumor cells. This and other evidence strongly suggests that an individual's performance in the face of the malignant situation varies. Some of us are far more resistant to cancer than are others.

Despite this immunologists are not prepared to accept the theory that when cancers take hold and spread an *a prori* failure of the immune system is responsible. Dangerous cancers can occur in anyone and escape immunological attention because of the extremely poor display of cancer and self antigens on their surface. Besides, the immune response can be foiled by tricks that the tumor cells can generate.

The story of Jennifer's miraculous recovery is by no means unique, although such occurrences are unfortunately rare. When pathologists take some of the secondarily infected tumor tissue, as in Jennifer's case, they find that in the furious immunological attack on the bacteria, innocent lung tissue and not-so-innocent tumor cells in the area of the struggle have been killed. The cancer cells are caught in the biological crossfire.

Because of these observations, my unit became involved in deliberate attempts to mimic the circumstances surrounding Jennifer's cure. Once a cancer in the lung had been localised with computer-assisted imaging, we injected some dead tubercle bacilli (the bacteria that when alive can cause tuberculosis) into the middle of the cancer. We had immunised the patients with this preparation two weeks earlier. A reaction occurred in the tissue with T cells pouring in, but the battle we had hoped for did not occur. In some ways that we do not understand the tumor was able to manipulate the immune response in that area so that the T cells that came in were 'turn off' not 'turn on' cells. That is why Jennifer's story is so unusual. She could get killer cells into her tissues when the bacteria invaded. Most cancer patients cannot.

To summarise: our immune systems are capable of recognising cancer cells in most tissues most of the time. They do this constantly as malignant cells frequently occur in our bodies. Suppressing our immune system markedly increases our risk of getting cancer. Some people are better at handling cancer immunologically than are others. Some tumors are much harder to detect than are others; they could fool anyone's immune system. They may be very hard to kill as they either do not display telltale surface antigens needed to excite our cancer killing cells, or they hide their antigens or suppress the immune system around the tumor-activating suppressor (turn off) T cells. Cancer is a formidable foe.

Following are some interesting and useful facts about different types of cancer.

Breast cancer will be diagnosed in more than one hundred and twenty thousand women in the USA in any one year. For women between their thirty-fifth and forty-fifth year, it will be the major cause of death. The incidence is highest in Caucasian women and lowest in women from the Indian tribes. The incidence is similar in most Western countries but lower in the East. Oriental women who move to the West assume the risks of other women living in that area. The causes of these differences are unknown.

The risk of dying of cancer of the breast becomes greater with each year lived, except for an unexplained plateau around fifty years of age. Women whose periods started early in life or ended after the age of fifty-five are at greater risk that women with a more typical menstrual history.

Irregular periods are associated with an increased risk of cancer. If a woman has her first child after the age of thirty, her risk is three times that of a woman who has her first baby at eighteen years of age.

This form of cancer does tend to run in families. If a woman has a mother or a sister who develops breast cancer, she is three times more likely to develop this cancer than if she did not have this familial incidence. This risk is heightened further if a woman had a sister who developed cancer before menopause.

Other factors that increase the risk are diets high in animal fats, obesity and radiation to the chest in the form of X-rays and atom bombs. There was a marked increase in breast cancer among Japanese women who survived Hiroshima.

Prevention is definitely the best approach to this form of cancer. Ninety per cent of women find their own cancer but too often their discovery is accidental. Regular, skilled self-examination is the proven best weapon. Women after their fortieth year who belong to a high-risk category should have X-rays of their breast (mammography) annually as this is a reliable tool for most women and can now be done with extraordinarily low doses of radiation.

Many women with breast cancer have malignant cells with membranes on which are receptors for the female sex hormone estrogen. This hormone, once bound to that receptor, stimulates the growth and spread of these highly malignant tumors. Drugs that block interaction of the hormone and the cancer cell are proving very worthwhile.

Technology has been developed to readily tell whether a patient's particular tumor cells are using sex hormones for growth or not. Anti-estrogen therapy can be given if the cells are dependent on this hormone and, if that fails, more drastic measures such as the removal of ovaries in pre-menopausal women and the little adrenal glands that sit on top of the kidneys can follow. The ovaries and the adrenal glands both produce sex hormones.

For small tumors diagnosed early, surgery or radiotherapy are recommended. For tumors that are spreading, more radical surgery may be needed together with radiotherapy, anti-hormone therapy and cancer-killing (but very toxic) drugs. With local tumors, survival rates five years after diagnosis may be expected to be between 40 and 80 per cent. Even with the best available treatment, a 10 per cent survival rate of five years is all that could be expected for cancer that has spread beyond the breast.

Today, breast cancer is managed better than ever before but it is still a major health hazard for women (and also for 900 men per year in the United States). One can only end this section by urging every woman to be ever vigilant and thoroughly trained in the best methods of breast self-examination.

Lung cancer

For reasons we have mentioned earlier, no cancer is more distressing to discuss than lung cancer. The disease would all but disappear if people would *stop smoking*. In the USA, more than one hundred thousand men and fifty thousand women develop this malignancy each year. The incidence is rising dramatically in women, who are tending to smoke more at a time when men are smoking less. It is tragic that any graph showing the rising incidence of lung cancer and breast cancer in women demonstrates that the title of leading cancer killer of women will change in the next few years, with lung cancer becoming the most common form of fatal malignancy for women.

Death rates from lung cancer for both sexes are doubling every fifteen years. For men over the age of thirty-five, this scourge is the leading course of death by cancer. Most cases occur between the age of fifty-five and sixty-five years, but thousands of thirty-five-year-olds die from lung cancer every year.

Perhaps the most sobering statistic for those few readers who will still smoke, having read the earlier parts of this chapter, should be this: at the time of diagnosis the disease is incurable in 70 per cent of cases. Survival of five years with this form of cancer is achieved by only 8 per cent of patients.

Lung cancer is, in reality, bronchial (airway) cancer and it starts when cancer-causing agents are inhaled into the airways. The cancer develops slowly but symptoms associated with this growth develop even more slowly. Sixteen per cent of patients are diagnosed as having lung cancer by a routine chest X-ray; the majority of other patients present themselves after coughing up some blood or because they have developed a nasty cough. As we have said, it is too late for a cure in 70 per cent of these cases.

Most patients with lung cancer are immunosuppressed by the disease and that, of course, facilitates its spread. We have excellent evidence that smoking, apart from stirring up oncogenes, disturbs the normal surveillance mechanisms found in the airways and for this reason smoking is a double hazard.

Apart from smoking, the only other numerically significant cause of lung cancer is asbestos. Chronic inhalation of asbestos particles into the lungs can cause the disease in an alarming percentage of exposed individuals. For this reason there is a massive effort in most countries to make sure that asbestos, used as a fire retardant in so many buildings, is completely covered. Unfortunately many cities have ordinances that demand the removal of all asbestos from public buildings. The perform-ance of this work is extremely hazardous and may cause many more problems than would occur if the asbestos was left alone and very good maintenance techniques were pursued to prevent its fibres leaking into the air.

Bowel cancer

Roland was fifty-six years old when his bowel habits changed. He had always had a tendency towards being constipated; now he was noting frequent days when his stools were, for him, surprisingly loose. He felt well and was not unduly distressed about the symptom. About two months after the onset of his changed bowel habit he put on a pair of pants and realised that he had lost a significant amount of weight; they looked decidedly baggy. He was puzzled. His appetite was good and he felt he was eating as much as ever. Still, he did not think the situation warranted a trip to his family doctor.

Three months later he was still losing weight and had some discomfort in the lower part of his belly; not serious, but nagging. It was the blood he passed one day with his stool that finally fired off alarm bells in his brain. His doctor could feel the cancer in his rectum with his finger, so low in the bowel had it developed.

To give him a fighting chance, his rectum was removed by a surgeon who simultaneously diverted his bowel away from his rectum, so that it could empty through an opening made in the skin of his abdomen (a colostomy), but all too late. The cancer had spread to his liver and he died within a few months.

Cancer of the large bowel and rectum is one of the commonest forms of the disease. In the USA 5 to 6 per cent of all men and women will develop this tumor. The incidence of this form of malignancy and the survival of patients after surgery has not improved in the last forty years. Newer approaches such as immunotherapy are promising and much needed.

The major and appropriate effort being made at this time concerns the identification of substances we eat that may cause cancer, foods that we could eat that might prevent cancer and ways of protecting the bowel from dangerous chemicals. Other urgent matters that need pursuing include ways of screening the entire population over fifty years of age for early cancer and the identification, for closer scrutiny, of those individuals who have a higher than normal risk of developing cancer.

A most fascinating and potentially useful observation has been made by scientific studies of bowel cancer in Africa. Where fibre content in the diet is high and stool bulk accordingly large, there is a much lower rate of cancer than is found in areas where little fibre is consumed. The theory that has been generated (but awaits formal proof), suggests that fibre (wheat bran and fibre from citrus fruits are the best sources) increases the bulk of non-absorbable waste in the bowel which understandably wishes to get rid of it. Transit time through the bowel is therefore hastened. Potential cancer-causing chemicals that may have been ingested are not allowed to linger and communicate with oncogenes. There is also some evidence that some chemicals with the potential to cause cancer are actually bound to fibres and eliminated from the body with them.

Whilst on the matter of diet, there is no doubt that high fat diets (containing, particularly, unsaturated fat) increased the risk of colonic cancer. In Japan, cancer of the bowel was an extremely rare disease until they adapted the bad eating habits of the western world. As their cholesterol shot up, so did their incidence of bowel cancer.

One of the more relevant and interesting observations of late concerns the geographic clustering of cases of bowel cancer in areas where the trace element selenium is lacking in the soil. It would be a wonderful break if adding selenium to our diet (just like adding fluoride to our water for teeth) prevented or minimised the incidence of bowel cancer.

If the entire population could be screened annually for cancer of the bowel the occurrence of the incurable form of the disease would all but disappear. Unfortunately, this is not economically feasible, even in Western countries. Unlike lung cancer, this form of cancer grows slowly. Between the start of the cancer and the development of symptoms, and certainly before its spread, a period of two to five years elapses. If cancer is detected by a routine examination, i.e., before symptoms develop eighty to one hundred per cent of patients are cured by simple surgery. The question thus is, how do we screen populations for this problem?

First let us identify groups at highest risk. To start with, we must say that everyone over forty years of age is at risk (one in twenty-five will develop this form of cancer in the Western world). Those patients with inflammatory bowel disease such as ulcerative colitis have a higher risk. Strangely, women who have had breast cancer or genital cancer have a considerably higher risk of developing bowel cancer than women who have not had these problems. Patients with little protrusions from the bowel wall called polyps are at risk and should be watched carefully. People with this cancer in the family have a four times greater chance of getting the disease.

Having identified high risk groups, how do we screen them for cancer? The most promising technique for mass screening utilises hemoccult (hidden blood) cards. These cards are impregnated with a chemical substance exquisitely sensitive in detecting blood in stool even if it is present in only trace amounts. If every person were to regularly test his or her stool for the presence of microscopic amounts of blood, thousands of lives could be saved. Not that the test is foolproof by any means. Not all cancers bleed while they are curable. What is important, of course, is that the majority do. Patients must refrain from eating meat, chicken and fish for twenty-four hours before they test their stool and they are advised to eat a lot of roughage during the period before testing to make it more likely that an early cancerous lesion will be irritated and bleed.

Despite the problems associated with this test, at least 50 per cent of patients with positive tests have cancer, and 86 per cent of those people have curable disease, which indicates the importance of pushing on with research into this promising approach.

Apart from hemoccult cards, the detection of cancer requires an examination of the bowel itself. All in the high risk groups mentioned above may like to discuss with their doctors the usefulness of having an examination of the bowel with an X-ray and/or sigmoidoscopy every two years or so.

Remember, bleeding, change in bowel habits (constipation or diarrhoea), lower belly discomfort, nausea and vomiting, and weight loss are the symptoms of bowel cancer.

Cervical cancer

Issa Bella is a tall and once-beautiful woman of the Pearl tribe of West Africa. She is twenty-four and works as a prostitute in St Louis, a pathetically poor but populous city on the coast of west Africa north of Dakar. To find clients, she mainly works the dance halls around the town which are extremely popular night spots, as West Africans love to dance and do so extraordinarily well. One is particularly appreciative of their skills when one listens to the difficult rhythms they prefer. Issa Bella had been working since she was fifteen years old. West Africans age rapidly, but this chronologically young women was ageing even more rapidly than is usual in this part of the world. She could even have passed for someone of forty years in the West.

Her remarkable French doctor introduced me to Issa Bella when I visited St Louis while working in Dakar. Marcel, the doctor in question, and his wife Lisette ran a blood bank and clinic for patients with sexually transmitted diseases. Marcel was alarmed at the amount of cancer involving the cervix that he was seeing in young African women, particularly the prostitutes. Here was Issa Bella at twenty-four years of age with a large malignant ulcer on her cervix. Marcel was convinced that cancer of the cervix was being caused by a virus that was presented to the genital tract during intercourse.

A few anatomical details are needed at this point. Around the entrance to the womb (uterus) is a small very muscular passageway. This guardian of the inner sanctum is the cervix. It keeps things in the uterus that should be there (such as babies) and lets things out that should be let out (such as the menstrual flow). The cervix projects downwards into the vagina like pursed lips. As such it is very much in communication with anything that comes into the vault of the vagina. The cervix is lined by a delicate membrane of cells that often become malignant, giving rise to the condition known as cervical cancer.

Issa Bella, already in her tenth year as a prostitute at the age of twenty-five, took no precautions. She had suffered numerous and repeated sexually transmitted diseases. She was very poor despite being busy; prostitutes charge only between forty cents and one dollar in these small towns where the competition is fierce. She certainly could not afford to use the pill.

She had had two pregnancies; her first child miscarried, her second was born and welcomed into her family but died of malaria at the age of two. The period following the second pregnancy had been a rough one for Issa Bella. Her uterus became infected and the Fallopian tubes were seriously damaged, effectively sterilising her. Now at twenty-five she had a horrible cancer in her cervix. Marcel thought correctly, that such a woman could be a valuable subject for a research project that would attempt to investigate the cause of cervical cancer.

For many years epidemiologists have been saying that the risk of developing cervical cancer is markedly increased in any woman who begins her sexual activity at a young age, and is directly related to the number of sexual partners experienced.

You may remember from the chapter on pregnancy that seminal fluid has properties that can suppress immune responses around the cervix. It is possible that seminal fluid could blunt such an attack by T cells trying to pick off cervical cells that have just become malignant. Certainly cancer in this region is practically unknown among women such as nuns who lead sexually inactive lives.

However, the more likely explanation, and one that would encompass the risks associated with promiscuity, would emphasise that the more sexual partners a woman has, the greater are her chances of being exposed to sexually transmitted viruses such as the herpes virus or another that has been incriminated recently, the papillomavirus. Certainly the virus that causes genital herpes and is sweeping the world, the herpes simplex virus Type 2, is more commonly found in the cervix of women with cancer than in others.

This form of cancer is very prevalent in women of Latin America and Africa. This cancer is more prevalent among the socio-economically deprived of the world and in women who have had multiple pregnancies. Both factors are often related, of course. One warning that is now acted upon comes from studies showing that female children, born to mothers given female sex hormones during pregnancy, have a much higher incidence of cancer of the cervix than normal when they become adults.

Fortunately studies have clearly demonstrated that cancer of the cervix is not related to the use of a contraceptive pill.

Serious consequences of this cancer can be avoided by its early detection. Regular (every second year) 'Pap' smears (named after Dr Papanicolou who described the usefulness of this approach) in which a scraping of the cells from the cervix is examined microscopically to look for malignant changes, will prevent incurable disease developing unnoticed. If the cancer does develop it will announce itself with small amounts of bleeding after intercourse, a discharge or heavier-than-usual monthly bleeding. The American Cancer Society looking at the cost-benefit ratio of Pap smears has recommended that women twenty years of age or older, but with no symptoms, and those under twenty, who are sexually active, have a Pap smear annually for two consecutive years and at least one every three years until the age of sixty-five. Women at higher risk should have yearly smears.

Melanoma

Our skin is a truly miraculous organ. Not only, as was pointed out in the Allan Sherman song, does it 'keep your insides in', but it acts as a primary defense against infection. Unbroken skin allows inside only what it wishes to allow inside.

Unless you happen to have black skin, there is no doubt that you are foolish if you deliberately expose your precious skin to the rays of the sun. Skin, as opposed to its owners, hates sunlight. It shrivels and cracks, ages and protests but still more and more people expose more and more skin to the sun. Dermatologists find tanning to be offensively ugly; how can people deliberately spoil something as perfect as unexposed skin?

The most serious consequence of exposing skin to sun is a particular form of skin cancer known as melanoma. Here, under the carcinogenic influence of sunlight, pigment cells in the skin have oncogenes activated and a tumor that is arguably the most dangerous of all cancers is born. All the cells in the skin are rapid dividers even when healthy; skin cancers can multiply and spread very rapidly.

Harmless pigmented 'growths' on the skin are called moles, and many people have hundreds of these tumors scattered around their surface. The fact that we are used to seeing pigmented spots on our skin may make us fail to notice the arrival of the cancerous variety.

In the Western world, the incidence of deadly melanomas has doubled in the last ten years and shows no signs of slowing. If you are fair skinned, have blue grey eyes and expose your skin to the sun in bursts (the weekends-only exposure at the beach habit), you are at most risk of developing this lesion.

This cancer responds very poorly to even the most potent anticancer drugs, and laughs off radiotherapy. Some melanoma can spread to every corner of the body and are then incurable; early recognition followed by surgical excision is the only worthwhile strategy. This should be easy, as the cancer is there for all who look with an informed eye to see. Melanoma is a medical emergency and removal as quickly as possible is essential.

This is a tumor that our immune system can recognise and spontaneous cures do occur, but all too infrequently. Horrible sight or not, we should all inspect all of our skin frequently to look for the following 'telltale' signs that should have us running to our doctor's office.

- Any pigmented spot on your skin that has either an irregular border or a lack of uniform color (that is, has more than one shade noticeable) must be removed. The important colors that are signs of malignant melanoma include shades of red, blue or *white*. Cancerous lesions can be uniformly colored and then they are usually bluish black, bluish grey or bluish red. These must be removed.
- Any pigmented spot that changes significantly and rapidly in size or color or bleeds must be removed.
- A spot that becomes itchy or painful must be removed.

Chances of surviving from melanoma can be assessed by examining the thickness of the cancerous tissue once it has been removed surgically.

Males and females who have a poor degree of tolerance to sunlight (i.e, who develop sunburn after even short exposures to the sun and who tan poorly), have a very high chance of getting melanoma and should not take the risk. In the long run they will not enjoy the results of repeated sunning anyway.

More women than men get melanoma, but it spreads faster in men. Melanomas developing on the chest, back or abdomen tend to be worse than those developing on the arms or legs. Detected early, the cure rate for melanoma is 80 to 100 per cent. With any spread, however, only 10 per cent of patients will be alive five years from diagnosis. Immuno-therapy, as we will see, may add significantly to our ability to obliterate this cancer.

The treatment of cancer

We live in an age when purveyors of alternative medicine advertise blatantly that they can cure cancer with everything from apricot pits to caffeine enemas. This is a particularly tragic form of fraud, as it preys upon the fears of those people with extensive cancer who cannot be helped by the currently accepted strategies of the medical profession. Medical Science seems close to improving our ability to manage many forms of cancer, and it must be stressed that great strides have already been made with the conventional approaches to the treatment of cancer now to be described.

Surgery can be curative and therefore the best approach to tumors that are accessible to skilfully wielded scalpels is removal. If the cancer has not spread beyond the area excised surgically, then treatment of it can be expected to be 100 per cent successful. The best chance of a surgical cure occurs in those cancers that announce their presence early in their development. Skin, breast, stomach, bowel and uterine cancers are some of the tumors that can be cured by surgery if detected early enough. For this reason there is an understandable emphasis in preventative medicine, on regular checks for early symptoms and signs of malignancy. Even if surgery is not curative it is often best to remove the bulk of the tumor so that it will not interfere with a local and vital function, by, for example, obstructing the bowel. After removal of the main mass of the tumor other 'mopping up' procedures can be used.

Sometimes the new machinery available for the delivery of radiotherapeutic beams can deliver sufficient radiation with such precision that this form of therapy can be curative and, indeed, may be the first line of therapy. Often, however, radiotherapy is used for palliation; slowing the growth of a tumor and reducing the pain associated with an infiltrating growth that is eroding sensitive nerves.

Radiation destroys cancerous (and normal) cells by damaging their chromosomes. As a result they lose their ability to divide. When they attempt to do so they become so genetically disorganised that they die. The more rapidly a mass of cells is trying to divide, the more sensitive will that mass be to the effects of radiation.

Major problems associated with radiotherapy include getting enough radiation to the tumor without damaging surrounding tissues and, even more importantly, protecting vital healthy tissues, such as bone marrow, as even small amounts of irradiation could damage delicate young cells necessary for our survival. You will remember that the bone marrow is responsible for the production of red and white cells (with the exception of T cells) and the clot promoting cells known as platelets.

The final conventional approach to the management of cancer utilises chemotherapy. Here we administer drugs either by mouth or intravenously and wait for these toxic chemicals to be delivered via the bloodstream to the tumor. The advantage of this approach is that in most cases it should be possible to get the drug to every cancer cell in the body. The problem is that normal cells in all tissues will be exposed to the toxin as well as the cancer cells. Hence, scientists have developed a collection of cellular poisons preferentially taken up by cancerous cells.

There are cells in our body that quite normally divide rapidly but, unlike cancer cells, do so in a controlled fashion. Normal or not, the drugs used to kill rapidly dividing cancer cells will penetrate these normal cells and kill them. The cells lining the intestinal tract and bladder, the cells in our bone marrow and the hair follicles are some of the most frequently affected normal cells. If you see children or adults attending a cancer clinic you cannot help but notice how many have lost their hair.

Chemotherapy can cure some forms of cancer, especially some forms of childhood leukemias, but most often chemotherapy produces a remission (freedom from symptoms) for variable lengths of time and in that way prolongs life. The art of the chemotherapist is to prolong life which has an acceptable quality. All chemotherapists long for the day when their skills will no longer be needed.

To-day, as we have discussed in the chapter on transplantation, our ability to perform marrow transplants allows us to push chemotherapy further than ever before. If the patient's marrow is unavoidably damaged in poisoning the cancer cells, then rescue is available, if risky. Ultimately, however, chemotherapy is not the solution to the cancer problem. What is? Certainly immunomanipulation holds the most promise at this time, and it is this that we will now discuss.

We now believe that cancer is perceived by Nature to be a threat to the species when it occurs (as unfortunately it does all too often) in the very young. Cancer was designed by Nature to develop in the elderly. We wind down our immune activity in later life and the incidence of cancer soars; all very orderly. Before it is cancer time, however, our immune system can and does protect us in a number of ways.

While we know a good deal about cytotoxic T cells, K and NK cells (discussed earlier) we have recently become intrigued by the observation that most, if not all, T cells, no matter with what antigen they are preoccupied on a day-to-day basis, can be activated to attack malignant cells. It is as if measles-recognising cells, together with all their brothers, have a second instruction delivered to them in the thymus, to kill measles virus or whatever they have been taught to recognise, but in addition, help out by joining in the attack on any cancer cell they may see.

What do all these T cells see when looking at cancer cells? We do not know. Observation is ahead of explanation at this point but the observations are worth understanding.

Imagine this situation. A man has a melanoma found on his chest, the surgeon removes it but studies show that the tumor has already spread to the man's liver. Unless the cells there are killed, he is doomed. Would that we could concentrate hard, summon up T cells and dispatch them to the liver to kill the melanoma cells! Our patient, unfortunately, shows no signs of doing anything immunological about his perilous situation.

If we take his all-too-complacent T cells out of his body and put them in an incubator with some interleukin 2, (the hormone-like agent T inducer cells secrete to activate killer T cells), the cancer-recognising property of the lymphocyte may well become active. After a few days in the incubator, re-infusion of these cells may have immediate and dramatic effects. The stimulated cells race like silver bullets to cancer cells in the liver and kill them.

We do not know if this phenomenon, induced outside the body by interleukin 2, occurs naturally in healthy people and whether this stops them from getting cancer. Such may be the case, but the phenomenon described and so clinically useful could be a totally artificial one. In favor of the latter concept are observations that the administration of interleukin 2 to patients in an attempt to make their cells kill cancer cells, is not successful as the doses needed to achieve this are too toxic. Of course, in the normally functioning body, very high doses of interleukin 2 may be effective and safely released only in those compartments where it is needed.

Thus it is that the observation that T cells, removed from the body and cultured with interleukin can kill tumors on reinfusion, has done two things. Firstly it has given us a potentially very valuable new tool to use against cancer. Research into the machinery needed for removing large numbers of T cells and safely culturing them for days and then returning them to a patient is well advanced and clinical trials well under way. Secondly, however, these observations require us to look at normal subjects and see if the actuation of most T cells against malignant cells is a natural phenomenon. If it is, we need to know what signal the cancer cell, presumably unwittingly, gives to trigger such a response. Another extraordinary property of these interleukin-2-stimulated cancer-killing cells is that they do not need to see self antigens before they kill.

This is well past the theoretical stage. Patients with melanomas, bowel cancers and tumors of the kidney, for example, who have cancer racing through their bodies have had it disappear after the reinfusion of their lymphocytes treated with Interleukin 2. To date we can say that in *some* there has been a relapse with time, in others no tumor is visible eighteen months after the completion of therapy. The potential of this approach is encouraging.

Another area of equal if not greater excitement in the immunotherapy of cancer world concerns the use of monoclonal antibodies to attack cancer cells. Let me explain in a not-too-fanciful story set five years hence.

Nancy looked at her chest X-ray as the immunosurgeon explained the situation to her.

'This white mass you can see here on the right side of your chest is cancer caused by your *pathetically* antisocial smoking habit,' he said. Nancy knew he was right, of course. No longer did nice people smoke, but she just couldn't help herself.

The surgeon continued, 'Look here, Nancy, the tumor has reached the stage where it has certainly spread around your body. Conventional surgery cannot cure you, but immunosurgery can.'

The surgeon skilfully removed Nancy's lung in much the same way as he would have done years before, but then the new technology took over. While an assistant closed up Nancy's chest, our surgeon left the operating suite and entered an adjacent laboratory. On a bench in this room was a cage containing eight mice; they would save Nancy's life.

Our immunosurgeon carefully cut some of the cancer tissue from the lung he had removed. He placed this cancerous material into a machine that disrupted the tissue into single cells, which were then washed in a special fluid that supplied them with nutrition. Our surgeon then drew up the cancer cells into a syringe, affixed a needle to its end and approached the cage of mice.

The mice got to work immediately, or at least their immune systems did. Lymphocytes raced into their skin to look at this obnoxious tissue newly placed there. Some cells looked at the cancerous cells and responded to the distinctive antigens they saw. B cells made antihuman antibodies and T cells geared up for an attack.

Other lymphocytes said, 'Airway tissue' and responded to the distinguishing antigens that they had recognised. B cells made anti-airway antibodies and T cells geared up for an attack.

But other lymphocytes recognised not only human airway tissue, but markers found only on cells developing in a malignant fashion. These markers were the product of oncogene activity and other genes that might have been activated. We know that no other cells in Nancy's body will have these markers; they may be Nancy and not totally foreign, but they are tumor-delineating. B cells made antihuman antibody and T cells geared up for an attack.

Two weeks after her operation Nancy was all but recovered from her surgery but was still faced with the need to get rid of the cells not surgically expiated. Two weeks after Nancy's operation, the mice had killed her tumor cells. Now living in their spleens, were B cells that had made and were still making antibodies to those differentiation antigens that distinguished Nancy's tumor cells.

The immunosurgeon returned at this stage and gently put the mice to sleep and removed their spleens. He put these organs in his tissue masher and single cells in the millions were harvested from the spleens of the mice. The cells were washed and placed in a test tube which was carefully sealed. At the end of this exercise, the immunosurgeon rested and held the tube up to the light. Too small to see with the naked eye were the spleen cells now resting in the nourishing liquid. Somewhere in there were B cells that could make antibody to Nancy's tumor.

Even under the most favorable circumstances, B cells will live only for a few days in a laboratory. How, then, will our new breed of cancer doctor find among all the millions of cells present in the test tube the particular B cells that can make antibody to Nancy's tumor, and nothing else? Even if a researcher finds them, how can he or she separate them and keep them alive long enough to get such little cells to make enough antibody for him to harvest it and inject it back into Nancy to kill her cancer cells? Easy, and in a way poetic justice; it will be done, thanks to the abilities of malignant cells themselves. Cancer cells will allow these mouse antibodies to kill Nancy's cancer.

Remember, we discussed the fact that cancer cells are immortal; put them into a test tube and feed them and they will live forever. Mice, like humans, get cancer of their antibody-producing cells (plasma cells). This form of cancer is called myeloma. When malignant plasma cells are put in a test tube inside an incubator, they live forever; not for four days, like the normal B cells. Plasma cells are factories that make antibodies; two thousand of them in every second. You will recall that individual plasma cells make only one antibody molecule; there is only one model produced by each of these factories. The antibody produced by *one* cell and its identical progeny (clones) is called a monoclonal antibody.

If you take a malignant cell and glue it with polyethyelene glycol to a normal but shortlived B cell, the genetic information that has been activated within that B cell moves across into the plasma cell. On its arrival there it activates these immortalised factories, which begin to produce massive amounts of the antibody that the B cell was trying to make.

By taking the B cells from the spleens of the mice that had successfully killed Nancy's lung cancer cells and then gluing them to cancerous plasma cells, an immortalised 'hybridoma' is formed that will produce buckets (literally) of antibody to the antigen or antigens the B cells had recognised as cancer-specific.

B cells from the friendly mice are glued to plasma cells. Each new cell is put in a little fluid in a separate compartment and allowed to continue multiplying. After a few days the immunologist and his team of helpers sample a little of the antibody being produced to see if antibody from a particular fusion reacts with Nancy's cancer cells, samples of which were kept at the time of surgery.

Hundreds of antibody samples from the various hybridomas are tested. A clone is found producing antibodies that will react to the differentiation antigen or antigens on Nancy's lung cancer cells. The cells producing this precious antibody are isolated and the rest discarded. Soon a large volume of fluid containing pure antibody is produced, that is, monoclonal antibody to something only displayed within Nancy's body on her cancer cells. When injected into Nancy, the antibodies will bind to these malignant cells and nothing else.

Now, if that were all, it would be a great story, but our immunosurgeon can do better than that. He knows that antibodies are specific but cannot kill cancer cells very well. They can find tumors better than anything else, but they cannot kill as well as can some other agents. Our immunosurgeon smiles as he prepares a poisonous antibody cocktail for Nancy's cancer.

Remember the tragic story of the ruthless terrorist who wished to dispose of a certain jumbo jet full of innocents? He gave his loving girlfriend a briefcase filled with explosives instead of the money he had promised her, instructing her to get on a specific plane. He then sat back and waited for his foul act to kill all the passengers, including his fiancee. All he required of her was that she should get on the correct plane; the explosives would do the rest.

Nancy's immunosurgeon had similar ideas and abilities to those of the terrorist just described. He called in his chemists, who took the mono-clonal antibodies that had been prepared against Nancy's tumor cells. Antibodies consist of long chains of amino acids with binding specificity at one end. To the other end they attached firmly, chemically, three killers.

The first to be locked onto the antibody was the toxin Ricin. This is the most powerful poison known to man; once it binds to a cell, that cell will die. This has been a famous poison ever since a KGB agent used it to kill a Bulgarian diplomat. The sharpened tip of an umbrella was dipped in Ricin and the unsuspecting fellow was jabbed in a crowd. He collapsed and died within seconds.

Besides the Ricin, the immunosurgeon asked chemists to couple some Chlorambucil, a highly poisonous anti-cancer drug, to the antibody. Some radioactive iodine was added. This isotope can be made so that it irradiates lethally but only for a very short distance of one to two cells. Now, the monoclonal antibody was ready to work. Here was an antibody that could recognise with exquisite accuracy Nancy's cancer cells, and *only* those cells. The antibody would deliver the three 'assassins' right to the target. No other cells would be victims; no cancer cells could hide.

Nancy was summoned and the mouse antibody, loaded with the cancer-killing agents, was injected into her veins. The treatment was repeated on consecutive days and, apart from a few shivers and chills, there were no side effects. The cancer cells died and Nancy was cured. To be super-cautious the plasma cells making the precious antibody were allowed to live. Should the cancer return, these same antibodies can be used again.

Fanciful story? Only a little. Monoclonal antibodies to differentiation antigens of human melanoma, breast, colon, ovary and lung cells have been made and used in humans. They have been tagged with chemicals and isotopes. Monoclonal antibodies labelled in this way have cured animals of cancer. We are only just beginning to develop our clinical expertise with humans. Nevertheless, it is quite accurate to say that the immunotherapy of cancer today is now a reality.

It is certain that the treatment of cancer will be revolutionised. Perhaps our immune systems are at fault when cancers develop; perhaps they are not. In either case it seems certain that our immune systems are only too willing to help us win this most important battle for a body very much at war.

6 | Dealing with AIDS

I
T is 1969. A ten-year-old black child walks across the rolling hills of the fertile plains near his village in the Mengo district of Uganda. Even the most casual observer can see that this boy is ill, wasted with the peculiar large belly of the severely malnourished. Very large lymph nodes have deformed his neck. He is limping. On his left foot is a reddish-brown nodule that is ulcerated and bleeding quite severely. It is obviously very painful. Other nodules of a similar nature, perhaps twenty in all, are on his body, although these are not ulcerated.

His mother has taken him to the tribal herbalist, who has tried a few different medicines. None has worked. The child's health is deteriorating and more purplish nodules have appeared on his skin. The tribal doctor is an experienced man and although he has never displayed to his charges the slightest doubt about his omnipotence, he knows his limitations. He has seen many similar cases recently and thinks that this child will probably not survive the summer. He informs the parents of the inherent wickedness of this child (which explains his inability to help) and tries to find a more suitable case for his talents.

The child, of course, is not wicked: rather, he is the victim of a terrible new disease spreading ever more rapidly across tropical Africa. He has been infected with a lethal virus that can destroy his immune system. Eighteen months earlier, he was given a blood transfusion after becoming very ill from a vicious attack of malaria. Many red blood cells were destroyed after his infection with this parasite and a severe anemia developed.

How could the tribal doctor know that the blood, given to the child, was donated by a man himself destined to die from the ravages of a virus circulating within the cells of his bloodstream? The ten-year-old child we

115

are discussing has subsequently had his immune system destroyed by this same virus. As a result, he has become an easy victim for a particularly nasty form of cancer known to us in the Western world as Kaposi's sarcoma (KS). This cancer showed in the skin of the boy as the purplish nodules already described.

Just what is Kaposi's sarcoma? Let us answer the question by starting at the beginning and meeting Kaposi, the man. In 1872, Dr M. Kaposi, a Hungarian specialist in skin diseases, wrote a paper that told a horrible story. He described in detail a young man who developed reddish-brown nodules, initially on his feet, which then spread to his hands and then, even more rapidly, over all his body. Kaposi commented on the peculiar sponge-like feel of these nodules and the fact that with time, as he stood by helplessly, the nodules, especially those on the patient's face, changed color, becoming bluish-red. His patient developed a hectic fever, lost weight and, as his strength failed, suffered bloody diarrhoea. He died coughing, drowning from blood-filled lungs. Kaposi organised an autopsy and as the internal organs of the dead man were exposed, the same reddish-blue nodules that peppered his skin were found to have proliferated in his liver, lymph nodes, lungs and many other sites. All Kaposi could do was report the strange facts to his colleagues.

For nearly eighty years of this century, Western physicians interested in cancer saw enough KS to come to one firm conclusion. The most aggressive and lethal form of this rare disease occurred in patients who were immunosuppressed; that is, a weakening of the immune system seemed to predispose them to the development of this form of cancer.

Thus KS was noted to occur in some patients who had had a kidney transplant. Such patients must be given drugs to poison their T cells so that they cannot reject their new kidney. The administration of these drugs must balance the risk of rejection against the risk of overwhelming infection. Infections are all too common when the balance is not quite right and in this setting a patient may develop KS or indeed other forms of cancer. Stopping the immunosuppressing drugs in such circumstances has sometimes been associated with recovery of the immune system, which is then capable of rejecting the cancer.

In the United States in 1981, only two cases of cancer among every 10,000 reported were cases of KS. While KS remained rare in the Western world, however, the aggressive form of this disease had become much more common in parts of Africa. Indeed, in the fifteen years prior to 1981 there was a tenfold increase in this form of cancer in many countries of Africa.

KS was appearing among the black population, with very few cases being reported in the Indian or white populations of countries such as Uganda. In its epidemic form, KS mainly attacked the young, most victims being under twenty years of age. We now know that during the

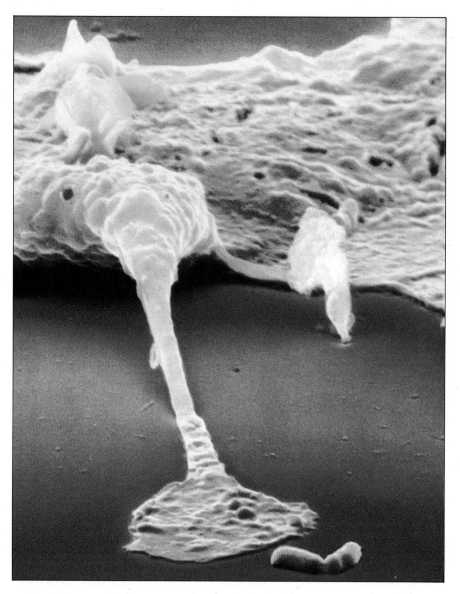

A macrophage (in this case an antigen presenting cell) reaches out for an antigen about which it is suspicious. The cell will pick up the bacterium and show it to an inducer T cell to determine whether it is self or foreign.

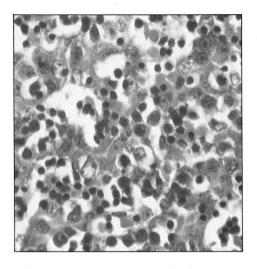

The cells of the immune system start life in the liver of the fetus. They are seen here as blue dots in a biopsy of liver from a 10 week old fetus. They will migrate to the thymus to be educated as T cells or to the bone marrow to become B cells.

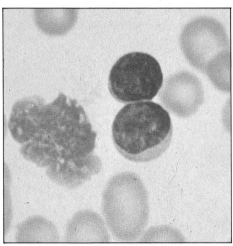

After education T and B lymphocytes circulate in the blood. The two round cells here are members of the immune forces. A B cell is floating on top of a T cell.

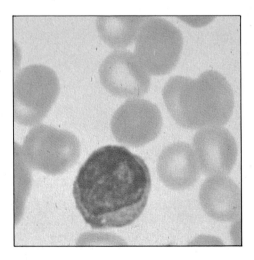

Before secreting antibodies B cells must recognise a specific antigen which will bind to some of the hundreds of thousands of identical antibody receptor molecules that cover its surface.

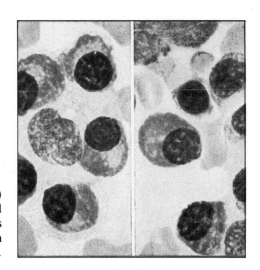

B cells that have recognised (bound) antigen turn into a factory that will produce and secrete 2,000 antibodies per second. The cells are now known as plasma cells.

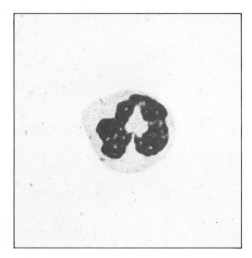

Antibodies activate those inflammation producing chemicals known as complement. They in turn activate these vital scavenger cells called neutrophils capable of swallowing and killing bacteria.

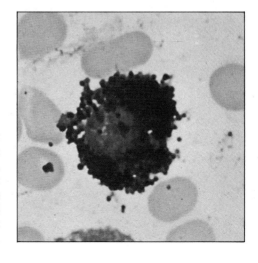

Immediate hypersensitivity or allergic reactions occur when allergens (grasses, dust, moulds, pollens etc.) bind to IgE on mast cells such as the one shown here which can release histamine and similar chemicals from the dark granules.

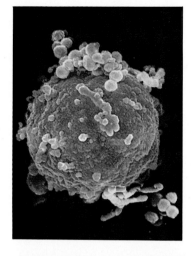

Left: A human B lymphocyte seen binding bacteria (coloured green) to surface receptors that allow that special cell to recognise this specific antigen. The cell will now divide to form plasma cells and secrete antibodies that can attack these bacteria.

Below: At a lower magnification, the ability of macrophages to extend their antigen trapping arms (pseudopods) is readily demonstrated.

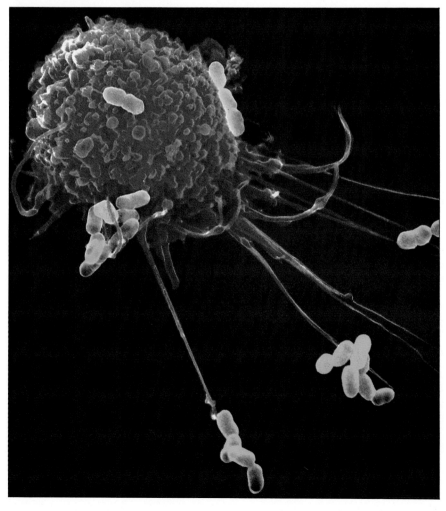

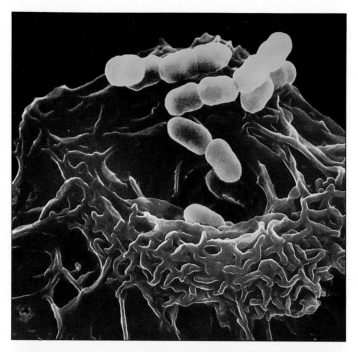

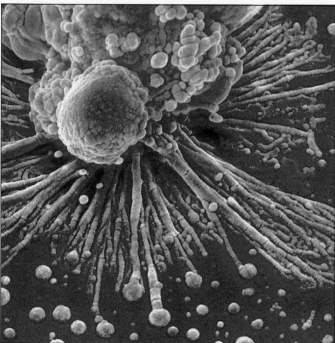

Top: Some macrophages are involved in swallowing and killing antigens. Here we see a macrophage activated by T cells or antibody on the green bacteria, actually swallowing bacteria one by one.

Below: An activated macrophage throwing out dozens of tentacle-like pseudopods to mop up globules of oil (yellow drops).

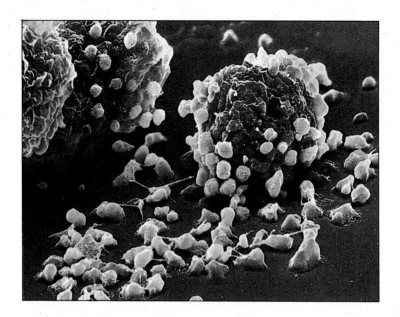

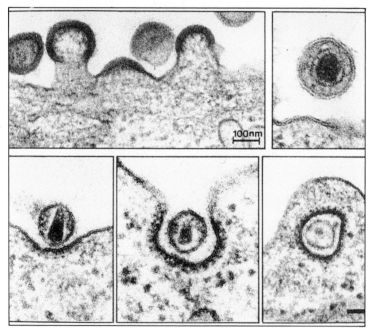

Top: A mast cell coated with IgE antibody has exploded after an antigen recognised by the IgE has landed on the surface of the cell. Tiny granules full of powerful chemicals like histamine are inside these granules. Twenty four per cent of us suffer 'allergies' when an excessive release of these chemicals affect blood vessels and the bronchial tree.

Below: The invasion of a T cell by HIV is illustrated in the bottom pictures. Moving from left to right the HIV can be seen binding to the CD4 molecule then being swallowed by the T cell. The top pictures, again moving from left right, show new AIDS virus budding out from the dying T cell.

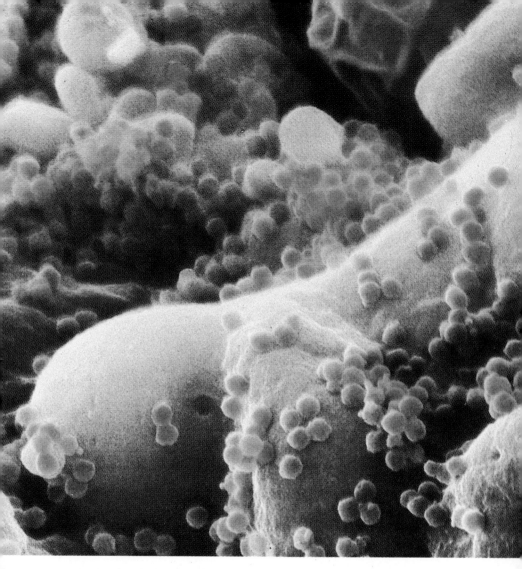

AIDS viruses escaping from a dying T cell and ready to move into new T cells and produce more damage to the immune system.

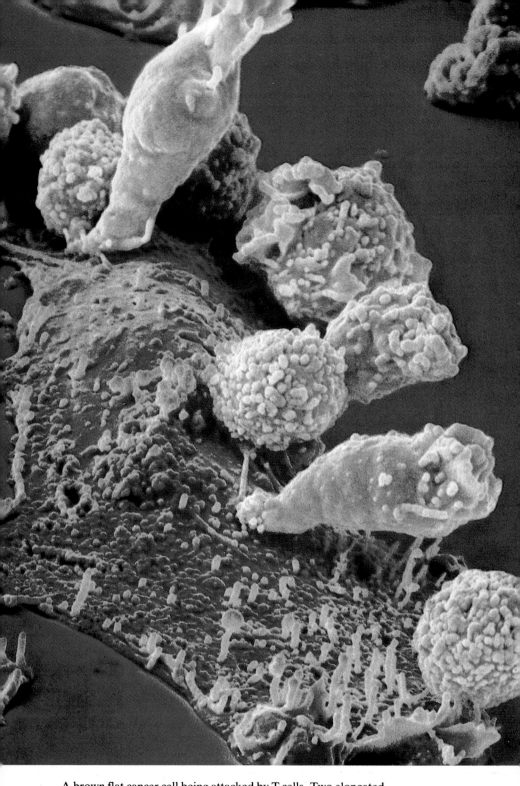

A brown flat cancer cell being attacked by T cells. Two elongated
T cells show blebbing and are dying; two others are alive and well, while
the cancer cell is almost dead.

early 1970s the disease was equally prevalent in Tanzania, Zaire and Angola and cut a path across the tropical girth of Africa.

Some doctors and missionaries asked why such a rare form of cancer, usually associated with severe immunosuppression (at least in the Western world) occurred so frequently in Africa. No one could answer the question; few people were really interested. At the time no one dreamed that the strange epidemic being reported was the start of the scourge now known as AIDS. Indeed, AIDS was discovered in the United States of America and only after much detective work were its origins traced back to tropical Africa.

At the Center for Disease Control (CDC) in Atlanta, Georgia, epidemiologists (medical detectives) and other specialists monitor, by means of reports coming to them from hospitals and doctors all over the country, the infections that trouble the population of the United States in any given week. In April of 1981, the scientists at CDC noted two strange reports, one from New York and one from Los Angeles. From each city cases were reported of homosexual men who had developed severe pneumonia caused by the organism known as *pneumocystis carinii.*

Pneumocystis carinii is a strange organism. It is neither a virus nor a bacterium but it belongs to a group of microbes known collectively as protozoans. We have already discussed some members of this family; such organisms cause malaria, African sleeping sickness and a disease commonly suffered by humans who live in close contact with domestic cats. *Pneumocystis carinii* is not one of the more powerful members of this family. It poses no threat to the normal immune system, whose T cells readily detroy this agent. It frequently takes advantage of immunosuppressed states, however, and then it can cause severe, even fatal, infection of the lungs. The organisms can often be found deep in the trachea or windpipe of normal humans, as if in taking up residence there they are hoping for an immunological disaster that may allow them to swoop down into the lungs where they may grow into tiny cysts (hence the name). The lungs of people infected by these organisms develop a severe pneumonia.

Within two months CDC had heard of many more cases all occurring in gay men. A number of these gay men had not only this peculiar form of pneumonia, but also Kaposi's sarcoma. The CDC now believes that the first two cases of AIDS occurred in 1978 and 1979 in the New York City area. Both cases involved gay men, who both developed Kaposi's sarcoma. Very rapidly physicians began to ask why two serious consequences of immunosuppression should be visited upon gay men.

The gay young men who were being reported as desperately ill with KS and severe penumonia had previously been reasonably well, with no known serious diseases. For lack of specific knowledge, it was said that they had *A*cquired an *I*mmuno *D*eficiency *S*yndrome (a syndrome is a collection of symptoms and signs that suggest an identifiable illness). Thus the term AIDS was born.

Now we know that AIDS is caused by a particularly dangerous virus designated, for obvious reasons, the Human Immunodeficiency Virus (HIV). With this information the pieces of the jigsaw puzzle seem easy enough to fit into a pattern but at the time that these first few cases were being studied in the United States of America, the matter was indeed most mysterious. Certainly nobody was linking the strange events being described on both coasts of the United States to any happenings in Africa.

As far as we know, the virus responsible for AIDS first caused problems for humans in Africa, beginning its invasion of the human population perhaps twenty or even thirty years ago. The basic facts are simple: the AIDS virus can destroy the immune system of an infected individual, who can then easily fall prey to such diseases as KS and *pneumocystis carinii* pneumonia (PCP). But where did this most destructive of viruses come from? How did it get from Africa to America? Why is it that in the United States, and at least initially in seventy-four other countries, it has mainly been a problem for gay men?

In order to approach the answers to these questions, we must realise that viruses continue to experiment rapidly and constantly. The results of their work may lead to what looks like the development of brand-new viruses. Such appearances, however, may be deceptive, for what we perceive as a new virus may in fact be no more than the latest in a long line of ever-improving models.

Our best information suggests that the virus that causes AIDS evolved from a series of less successful prototypes. We believe it evolved in Africa. Careful analysis of the structure of the virus that causes AIDS tells us that it belongs to a family known as retroviruses.

This family has numerous branches. We first realised that some members could cause illness when studying diseases in animals. Certain retroviruses were found to cause a nasty brain inflammation in horses, a degenerative brain disease in sheep and leukemia in cats. (Leukemia is a condition in which specific white cells in the blood, that is, those involved in defense, not oxygen transport, start to divide uncontrollably.) Much research time has been spent on cat leukemia, for it kills millions of much loved pets annually, and of course, a commercial vaccine would be extremely successful. From these observations we knew in the pre-AIDS era that retroviruses tended to attack white blood cells and/or the brain and tended to trouble mainly animals. Currently, overwhelming circumstantial evidence suggests that a retrovirus previously able to infect animals mutated so that it could infect and then kill humans.

Animal viruses do not usually trouble humans, and vice versa. As we saw when discussing parasites, all invasive micro-organisms have a favorite host, and within that host a favorite site at which they would prefer to take up residence. Dogs do not get the flu and humans do not get distemper (although both animals get something very similar). It is now widely accepted that an animal retrovirus in Africa found itself in some young immunosuppressed Africans who could not eliminate it with the ease with which an animal virus would be destroyed by a healthy human immune system.

The earliest known case of human infection with the HIV virus occurred in a Ugandan male. He was infected by 1965 but the date of his infection is unknown. Researchers screening blood stored for twenty five years, originally collected for hepatitis research, found HIV in one sample. If the virus started its march through Africa in Uganda, then the dreadful deprivations of the Amin regime, coupled to chronic disease, would have facilitated its passage. Indeed malnutrition and malaria seem very important co-factors and may well have contributed to a less-than-hostile environment for the animal virus, allowing it to mutate into a lethal problem for humans. We know that viruses can gain strength from a sojourn through individuals with low resistance, becoming wilder and more dangerous as they do so. Some of the HIV prototypes reached new strength that allowed them to infect even healthy humans.

How did the animal virus get into humans in the first place? Certainly ingestion of animal tissues, especially brain and blood that had not been adequately cooked, could have been responsible. There is excellent evidence to suggest that the immediate precursor of the AIDS virus in Africa could have infected certain monkeys and that humans bitten by such monkeys might have become infected with the virus. Monkeys are eaten and their blood drunk in a number of parts of Africa.

The Green monkeys of tropical Africa were found to be infected with a virus very similar to the AIDS virus now devastating humans. The virus causes no ill effects within the monkeys, however; could this be the virus that changed once it entered some immunodepressed humans? Another virus, closely related to the AIDS virus, infects monkeys in Guinea-Bissau and Cape Verde and does kill monkey T cells. Indeed, there are now five viruses isolated from the T cells of humans with AIDS that differ from each other minutely but significantly. All have been traced back to African monkeys. The first two discovered have been called HIV1 and HIV2. The others will undoubtedly be classified similarly. Ninety-nine per cent of the cases of AIDS around the world are caused by HIV1 (usually just referred to as HIV), but HIV2 is on the move. It has spread from Africa to Portugal and marched into Europe, reaching as far as Germany. At this writing, is has not reached the USA or the southern hemisphere. Dr Robert Gallo, the co-discoverer of the HIV virus, feels that many primate retroviruses will have mutated into organisms with the potential for causing AIDS. We already know that individuals unfortunate enough to be infected with two AIDS-causing viruses simultaneously die more rapidly than those infected with only one virus. There seems little doubt from recent research that at some fateful moment in biological history one or more of these primate viruses entered man and changed its characteristics, initiating a modern plague.

The Human Immunodeficiency Virus developed in Africa and stayed there for perhaps twenty to thirty years before turning up almost simultaneously in the Caribbean basin and in Belgium. How it got to the Caribbean and why it settled most obviously in Haiti is unknown. Speculations abound, ranging from the transport of the virus by Castro's troups returning from Angola, to the idea that poor migrant workers from Haiti imported the disease on their return from attempts to find work in Africa. There is no doubt that the virus was transported to Europe by visitors (mainly students) from former African colonies.

From the time the AIDS virus arrived in Haiti, probably early in 1978, the events leading to the establishment of the epidemic in the Western world are far clearer. As are many other infectious agents, HIV infectious particles are concentrated in the seminal fluid of infected men. It is thus easy for one human infected with HIV to infect another by exchanging sexual fluid. Quite definitely the virus was picked up by gay Americans visiting Haiti and subsequently transported to Manhattan's gay community and then, in an ever-accelerating fashion, to gay communities around the world. To understand the speed with which the infection spread and the magnitude of the epidemic that resulted, one must emphasise that two very significant developments, one biological and one social, coincided, indeed collided, and created a recipe for disaster.

We have already mentioned the arrival of the AIDS virus in Haiti with characteristics that determined its presence and viability in sexual secretions. It is also present in circulating blood; the relevance of this will shortly become obvious. The sociological event was the 'gay revolution' occurring in major cities such as New York and San Francisco and indeed many others around the world. This revolution led to a new sexual lifestyle that could not have been better designed to disseminate the virus.

While we need to explore these concepts in detail, let us recapitulate at this stage. A virus that could damage the immune system emerged among poor, malnourished and diseased Africans in the late 1960s and early 1970s. The virus was present in considerable quantities in blood and sexual secretions. It was confined to Africa for some time but then burst forth almost simultaneously into Europe and Haiti. From Haiti it was transferred by sexual activity to visiting gay Americans. They transported HIV back to the liberated sexual atmosphere of San Francisco and New York, and the Western epidemic began.

It is important to examine homosexuality as a co-factor in the dissemination of this disease. If AIDS continues to spread through the world's gay communities, the already horrendous death toll (more than sixty thousand at this time) will increase even more and hundreds of thousands of deaths will occur. For this reason scientists have had to draw aside the veil of privacy that usually surrounds people's sexual habits and place the intimate behaviour of gay men under the microscope in the hope that they may learn more of the way that AIDS is spread. Prevention strategies require this knowledge.

We obviously need our sophisticated defense mechanisms in top condition if we are to win our battle against the microbial world. To ignore good nutritional advice and to eat so poorly that we deprive our defenses of the nutrients they need will certainly lead to immunosuppression and an increased risk of infection. Similarly, it is unquestionably dangerous and, yes, unnatural to repeatedly drug our bodies and introduce seminal fluid, especially from numerous different sexual partners, into the intestinal tract.

These judgments have nothing to do with morality, unless you regard naturalness, in the sense of working with Nature, as the ultimate morality. It is an undeniable fact that even ignoring AIDS, health hazards are visited upon many in our society who, in seeking pleasure, involve themselves in activities that place them at risk of picking up serious infections and damaging their immune systems. Although the AIDS epidemic has led many gay men to change their lifestyle, there is no doubt that their activities, flourishing in the late 1970s and early 1980s, represented a real hazard. While certainly the most significant, AIDS is only one of the numerous problems that can and did result. Let me state immediately that much of what follows applies equally to much heterosexual activity.

Seminal fluids can carry infections such as the hepatitis B virus, the cytomegalovirus that causes a mono-like illness or worse, bacteria such as those that cause gonorrhoea and chlamydia, the little spirochaete that causes syphilis and many fungi that can cause severe diarrhoea if allowed to enter the rectum. Last but not least, there is the ubiquitous herpes virus that infects at least twenty million Americans and may now be the most common sexually transmitted disease.

As millions of gay and straight folk can attest, genital herpes is bad news. Perhaps 20 per cent of the young population of the United States is infected with the herpes virus and the rate of infection is growing rapidly. Men and women can infect each other with this virus. A gay man whose anus becomes infected with the herpes virus suffers from extremely painful blisters in the area. The curse of herpes is that, in one out of every three victims, it does not go away after the first episode, but recurs at regular and not-so-regular intervals. Such unwelcome visits can continue for years. While fresh lesions are present intercourse is unlikely because of pain, but if after an attack sexual activity is resumed, the virus may still be present on the genital or rectal surface and ready to move on.

Pregnant women with genital herpes have a terrible problem. Sixty to eighty per cent of their babies will be infected if delivered vaginally. In babies, herpes infection can be fatal. When such a situation is discovered, the baby must be delivered by caesarian section.

The reason for discussing this now is to point out that very frequently sexual encounters with partners about whom one knows little or nothing are dangerous. Gay men with many different lovers have nearly all suffered from hepatitis B, syphilis, gonorrhoea, numerous bowel bacteria, fungi and anal herpes. They tend to socialise late into the night, smoke and use recreational drugs. Of course, a number also use hard drugs intravenously. The result of this lifestyle is that many gay men are chronically ill and may not have an immune system in tiptop condition should they be unlucky enough to come in contact with the AIDS virus.

It now seems certain that gay men from the United States who went to Haiti on vacation picked up the AIDS virus from sexual encounters with local men, many of whom sell themselves for money, as they are so poor. It is hardly surprising that, in cities such as New York, infection among the gay community spread rapidly. Most victims of the disease consider that they might have had between 500 and 5000 different sexual partners in their young lifetime. Thirty different sexual partners in one day is not uncommon.

Perhaps if we meet one of the young gay victims of AIDS and examine his story in detail, many of the major features of the problem will fall into place. James, lying pale and obviously exhausted in the bed, was only thirty-two years of age but looked twenty years older. He had recently lost his eyesight as a virus infected and destroyed his retina. As a result, his head moved constantly because he needed to localise the sounds reaching his ears. He tried to speak but even this required a physical exertion that made him breathless, causing his speech to be punctuated with gasps for air, despite the oxygen being fed into his nose. An organism had infected and destroyed most of his lungs.

His thirty pounds' weight loss of the last three months left him wasted and the skin under his arms, which had so recently been tanned and taut over strong young muscles, was pale and dry. Standing out from this pallor were numerous round purplish discolorations, some rising from the skin in discrete lumps. A careful examination revealed a similar lesion inside his cheek.

Cancerous cells developed in the blood vessels of this man's skin and were now multiplying and migrating out of control: KS. As he attempted to speak, his incoherence and removal from reality became obvious. Mercifully, this patient was only partially aware of his surroundings and situation. He had another organism which, finding no resistance from any infection fighting defence forces, had invaded his brain to produce the mental changes now so obvious.

We have been discussing the case of a sensitive and intelligent young lawyer. James's practice in a small law firm in middle Connecticut kept him busy during the week, but the weekends were his own. He was the second of three children. His older brother, married with two children, ran a small family business successfully. James had been an outstanding athlete at school. The youngest child, a sister, had just completed a degree in business administration and all seemed to be going well for this family.

If any of James's family knew that he was gay, and he thought his mother did, they never admitted it to him. In recent years James, a talented guitarist, had developed a preference for music rather than sport. He was thin and good-looking in a fragile way. He wore thick glasses which made him look more serious and scholarly than he really was.

He certainly did not dislike women. Once or twice he remembered being sexually aroused by a female. However, as early as his fifteenth year, he had realised that he felt the sensations so vividly and frequently described by his older brother much more frequently in the presence of men. By the age of sixteen he realised he could identify his sexual preference for men.

On one or perhaps many Saturdays between 1979 and 1981, he encountered once, or perhaps many times, the virus that would kill him. Being single and a professional, he was now able to encounter similarly orientated men in pleasant surroundings by visiting New York City. Here he considered his sexual adventures to be satisfying, civilised and safer than in earlier days.

In the past, he had sometimes felt passionate enough for sex with total strangers even in a toilet booth. But on this typical day things were very different. He drove to New York in mid-morning and entered a small, unremarkable-looking apartment building and walked up three flights of stairs with ease. He was fit and excited.

The top floor of the building had been converted into what at first looked like an executive-type health club. After using his key to enter the area he was greeted by the familiar sound of male laughter, the hectic sounds of splashing as arms propelled bodies through chlorinated water and the humid, in fact quite steamy atmosphere of this sunny area into which he strode confidently.

Around the perimeter of the room were perhaps twelve dressing rooms containing lockers and a comfortable chaise for private resting.

Louvred wooden doors provided access to these rooms. There were no locks on the doors. Most of the men in the room were naked; a few wore abbreviated shorts or swimming trunks. This was no collection of young gods of fitness, however; all shapes and sizes and a wide range of ages were represented. James guessed from a quick survey of the scene that he knew at least 50 per cent of the people present. He moved to a vacant dressing room where he changed into swimming trunks.

His first lover that day was an old friend with whom he had experienced sex on many occasions and they moved into the privacy of one of the dressing rooms for their encounter. Others, less inhibited, enjoyed each other while lying by the pool. It is certainly of more than prurient interest that in this first sexual session he not only kissed his lover on the mouth, but he took his lover's penis and semen into his mouth, and that he kissed with his tongue his lover's anus. It is almost certainly of deadly interest that before the day was over James would have four more sexual encounters, two with strangers, men he had never seen before that day.

During the day he was reminded of a problem he had been facing for two years. James suffered from genital herpes, tiny blister-like sores situated near his anus. They were not at their worst, but nevertheless they were painful. To receive the penises of his lovers into his anus, he used a lot of cream for lubrication to minimise the pain. He used a cream containing cortisone which he had bought without a prescription from his pharmacist.

During these passionate encounters this day, he experienced a number of orgasms. With each of these experienced lovers, he had time, as the moment approached, to break open a small capsule containing the drug amyl nitrite which he inhaled through his nose. The drug made his whole body flush with a warm felling and when he timed it right this feeling coincided with his orgasms; the intensity of the pleasure was wonderful.

During the sexual highlight of the day one of his lovers, to increase further the pleasure he was experiencing, twisted and pushed his fist into James' well-lubricated anus. He felt pain from the intense stretching that occurred and some of the delicate tissues around the anus tore, causing him to bleed a little, but he willingly accepted this pain because his sexual pleasure far outweighed the physical discomfort involved. By the end of the day five different men had discharged their sexual fluid into his rectum and he had returned the favor for three of them.

James showered and washed himself meticulously, as did the others present. He returned to Connecticut well satisfied with the pleasures of the day, already anticipating further encounters with these men, especially those he had met for the first time. He wished that Robert, the man with whom he had lived for four years, would come to New York and share these experiences with him. But Robert was not interested, did not like to experiment, did not wish to take drugs and simply wanted a quiet, monogamous life.

As James drove up the Connecticut turnpike, his thoughts turned to one of the men he had enjoyed that day. Passionate, certainly; performing normally, yes; but for all that, clearly not well. He was surely too thin, his eyes were dull. Had he imagined it, or was this man depressed? And then there was the matter of those two strange purplish red nodules on his hands. James had never seen anything quite like them.

Well, James is dead and Robert is dying and there can be no other conclusion than that James carried a lethal infection to his faithful partner.

A re-examination of James' activity on the day described above ilustrates some of the risk factors that contribute to the spread of the disease AIDS. The infectious agent capable of causing AIDS is present in sexual secretions. James took sexual secretions into his mouth and rectum. While skin is almost impenetrable and a superb barrier to infection while its integrity is unbreached, mucous membranes, those smooth, moist, filmy linings throughout the mouth and intestinal tract, are just the opposite; they are designed to facilitate the entry of materials into the vital areas of our body. These membranes in our intestinal tract absorb fluid and the nutrients from digested food. Viruses and many other infectious agents penetrate these linings easily. Nature was not foolish enough to leave these areas without protection and we have discussed earlier the special role of the secretory immune system. It is certain, however, that a number of organisms find that our inner skin provides an excellent route for invasion.

To absorb the nutrients obtained from a good roast dinner, the small intestine opens wide the blood vessels that flow into this area. As the blood vessels increase in size, more blood will flow through the area. As a result, there will be an increase in the temperature of all the cells around as metabolism is stimulated. Many of these cells will have their membranes stretched, opening tiny pores in the outer shell that will allow the nutritional factors that need to be absorbed and other matters to pass selectively from the intestinal tract into the blood. Once there, these nutrients may be whisked away for immediate use or stored in the liver.

The same increased blood flow and increase in the ease of absorption of chemicals (and, of course, an opportunistic virus) will occur after the use of amyl nitrite. This drug dilates blood vessels, giving that warm feeling that many feel adds to their sexual pleasure.

It does not take much imagination to see some risk factors for James. He may have taken infected sexual fluid from a man with AIDS into his mouth or rectum and then flushed open his blood vessels, facilitating the ease with which a virus or some other deadly micro-organisms might enter his body. When you realise that the surfaces of his mucus membranes were already breached by his genital sores and the traumatic nature of his lovemaking, it appears that James was actually inviting the deadly guest to come inside. The cortisone cream he and many gay men used as an anal lubricant before intercourse would not have helped local defense mechanisms, as cortisone can suppress the immune system.

So, what have we? A new virus, potentially lethal to humans, lives in Africa for some time then rapidly moves to Haiti then into the gay populations of the United Sates. At this point we know that the virus is in seminal fluid and enters the body of homosexual victims through the intestinal tract. If the virus can then be transmitted sexually to males, what about women?

I knew that American women would not be exempt from the curse that is AIDS very early in the AIDS story. Soon after we started our clinic and research into the disease at Yale, I met an extraordinary couple who performed a terrible and conclusive experiment.

Jane and Barbara were lesbians who had been living together in northern Connecticut for three years. The relationship seemed satisfactory to them, and they assured me it was stable. The couple's biggest frustration in life was their inability to have a baby ('to make our marriage normal') and in this department, but no other, they were willing to admit that men were useful. As adoption was out of the question, they came up with a solution that was common, they assured me, among lesbian couples.

Jane and Barbara knew many gay men. They started looking for a suitable genetic father for the baby that Barbara had decided to have (Jane, of course, would be the real father). Blue eyes and blonde hair were essential; they agreed on that much. Eventually they decided upon a beautiful young man named Tom.

Jane asked Tom whether he would help them get their much-wanted baby. He was bemused and flattered although, of course, he was not sexually interested. It was arranged that Tom would come to their apartment the following night, when Jane's research suggested Barbara's cycle would be at its most fertile, and masturbate into a dish. The seminal fluid would be aspirated into a small syringe and he was free to go.

Jane had learned that fertilisation was facilitated by meeting with sperm at the moment of orgasm. Therefore she took the syringe with Tom's semen into the bedroom and made love to Barbara. As Barbara's climax approached Jane inserted the syringe as far into her vagina as was possible and injected the seminal fluid. This exact scenario was carried out for six nights in a row, with Tom supplying the seminal fluid nightly.

He demanded and was paid $50 for his trouble on the last three occasions. Barbara did not become pregnant, but she was infected with the AIDS virus.

This case, of course, proved that when men are infected with the AIDS virus, vaginal sex places women at enormous risk of getting the disease. The AIDS virus must be able to penetrate the female genital tract and enter the body where it can do its damage.

Seminal fluid in the mouth, particularly if swallowed, must be presumed to be infectious, while seminal fluid ejaculated into the rectum of a woman is, from an infectious disease point of view, no less dangerous than it is for men.

After reading this story you will not be surprised to learn that in a number of countries around the world, women married to sterile husbands are turning to sperm banks for help. Collected sperm from the bank is artificially inseminated into the woman anxious to become pregnant and in many cases such attempts are successful. Many sperm banks pay for donations. Consequently, it is not unusual for money to be the main, if not the only, reason for a man providing some of his sperm. Sad to report, in recent years a number of donors have been infected with the HIV virus. As even the most careful history and examination of the donor could not have detected this situation, a number of sperm samples containing live AIDS virus were inseminated into women in many parts of the world. A number have gone on to develop the disease.

If men can infect men and men can infect women, what about the transmission of the virus from women to men?

Hermann was a German engineer working on a project for his company in the United States. The work would keep him in the northeastern section of America for two years. The construction job in which he played an important role was proceeding at a great pace and only once a year could he have time off from the project to return home for a few weeks. Hermann and his family had been through this deprivation before; similar projects had taken him to Asia and north Africa.

Hermann loved his three children and his wife. In sixteen years of marriage he had never dreamed of being unfaithful to her, at least not by *his* definition of the word. Sexual relief with prostitutes was quite another matter.

Sixteen months before I met him, Hermann had arrived in the USA and two months after settling in he had carefully chosen a prostitute. He always did it this way, he told me; find one you like, make sure she is clean and compatible, and stick with her. Regular customers get better treatment anyway. He knew that Priscilla, the girl he chose, was an intravenous drug addict, but weren't they all? He was certainly not about to get involved with the drug scene in any way.

He got on well with Priscilla, who was black; he liked black women. She introduced him to anal sex. He had six sexual encounters with Priscilla over a fourteen-month period. At the end of that time two things happened. In the few weeks before he saw me, Hermann had not felt very well. He had noted swollen glands under his arms and in his groin and he had experienced some drenching night sweats. He knew nothing of AIDS. Two days before coming to see me he had his last liaison with Priscilla and a terrible thing happened; she stole his wallet.

He felt betrayed, then very annoyed and with no sense of embarrassment called the police. They picked up a surprised Priscilla, who had the wallet in her bag, and off to jail she went.

Initially, of course, we did not know what was the trouble with Hermann but we had our suspicions. Sure enough, his T cells had the characteristic alterations that we see in people infected with the AIDS virus. Once the story was known we contacted the prison doctor, who was most co-operative, and Priscilla was sent down for us to check. She arrived in the clinic with her feet and hands cuffed (a little excessive, we thought), was tested and found to be infected with the AIDS virus.

Hermann decided to go home to Germany to await his fate. He lived for another two years. I only saw him once more six months later when he dropped into my clinic unexpectedly. He had returned from Germany, sick and all as he was, to testify against Priscilla. He had his own strict sense of duty. Priscilla had been out on bail and was sentenced to six months in jail but served not one day. She was released on medical grounds and disappeared. By this stage, of course, her medical condition was known; no one wished to deal with an AIDS victim in the local jail.

It is obvious from all of the above that it is a dangerous misnomer to refer to AIDS as the 'gay plague'; the AIDS virus has no sexual preferences at all. In the USA and many Western countries, the reservoir holding the virus was for some time locked away inside the gay community and members of it infected each other.

From the beginning of the AIDS story, however, the opposite has been true in Africa. Here most infections have involved heterosexual activities. The disease continues to spread at an alarming rate in this manner. Recent studies of the way that AIDS is creeping through Africa illustrates the great danger for the spread of the disease among heterosexual people in Western society if any significant reservoir of HIV builds up in that population.

Several million people in Africa are infected with HIV. At least twenty-four African countries are involved. Males and females are infected equally and 90 per cent have no identifiable risk factor apart from heterosexual activity. In countries where the question has been studied, patients infected with HIV have had an average of thirty different sexual partners while those who are not infected with the virus report a figure of four.

The infection rate among prostitutes is very high in many of these countries. Forty-three per cent of prostitutes are infected with HIV in

Rwanda, while even higher percentages are being recorded in Uganda and Kenya. In some studies, as many as 81 per cent of the prostitutes are infected and therefore could be spreading this disease. It is estimated that one infected prostitute could spread the disease to at least fifty of her clients in any given year.

One-third of HIV victims in Africa have had at least one other sexually transmitted disease and it seems likely that casual sex and the frequent use of prostitutes is responsible for most of the African cases.

Women in Africa appear to be more readily infected by men than those in some Western societies. It is considered likely that this results from the frequency of genital and cervical ulcers in malnourished and often diseased African women. Such ulcers would make it easier for the virus to penetrate mucus membranes and gain entry into the body proper.

After the AIDS virus arrived in New York and San Francisco and was identified as a sexually transmitted disease within the gay community, people rapidly realised that this was not the only way the disease could spread. To understand the next epidemiological bombshell that exploded AIDS out of the gay population, we need to look at how the AIDS virus causes so much damage to the immune system.

To avoid confusion I must explain why the virus that causes AIDS, the particular retrovirus we have been discussing for so long, underwent a name change. In the early days of the epidemic it was called the HTLV III virus. The name was inaccurate, but some might have read of the virus when this terminology was being used. The initials stood for *H*uman *T* Cell *L*eukemia *V*irus. Because it is called type III, there must obviously be types I and II.

Types I and II cause leukemia (cancer of white blood cells) in humans, though rarely. Type I causes a T cell leukemia and Type II a B cell leukemia, and a peculiar one at that. The B cells grow surface protrusions that under the microscope look like hairs, so that this form of leukemia is called hairy cell leukemia. Although both diseases are caused by retroviruses, they are not closely related to the virus that causes AIDS, though early research incorrectly suggested that a close relationship might exist.

When French workers trying to isolate the virus found the virus in the swollen lymph nodes of people infected with the agent that causes AIDS, they called it LAV; *L*ymphadenopathy (swollen lymph nodes) *A*ssociated *V*irus. To avoid confusion, scientists settled on the now universally accepted name HIV or Human Immunodeficiency Virus.

The HTLV I virus seems to have lived in southern Japan for 300 years or more, causing problems there, and only there, until late in the 1960s when it turned up in Jamaica, the United States and Israel and is now in most countries of the world.

When the HIV virus is implanted in the rectum, it attaches itself to the cells that make up the lining of the gut and passes through into the blood vessels lining the intestines. The passage of the virus may be facilitated by local injury. Some virus may go to local lymph nodes and stop there; other virus stays in the bloodstream.

How does the HIV virus destroy the immune system? The evolutionary changes that distinguish the precursor of the AIDS virus found in monkeys, from the HIV virus which infects humans, would seem to have been planned by some viral architect who knew his human immunology, so clever are the design changes incorporated. And yet in biological terms these apparently deserved triumphs are more like those of a man who, having no idea of a safe's combination, sits patiently twiddling the dials at random until suddenly he gets it right and the safe door swings open.

The right combination for the virus allows it to open a window in the membrane of the T 4 cell and march right in.

The HIV virus is surrounded by a coat or envelope constructed of specific proteins. One of these projects away from the surface of the envelope in the form of a probe. The physical shape of this probe is a mirror image of a protein known as CD4 on the surface of our alarm-sounding T cell. Such complementary structures make it possible for the virus and the T cell to 'dock', spaceship fashion. The HIV envelope probe acts as a key that can be inserted into a very specific lock on the membrane of a T cell. This form of intimate binding to the T cell's membrane activates mechanisms within the T cell which are programmed to take into the cell chemicals that have a right to know the combination. Usually these are nutritional elements. Unwittingly, then, T 4 cells swallow the enemy.

Never before has a virus that can be recognised or destroyed only if T 4 cells sound the alarm managed to give itself a survival advantage by directly attacking its enemy. Once safe inside the cell the coat around the core of the virus dissolves and the next phase begins.

The Human Immunodeficiency Virus carries all its genetic information in the form of RNA, a language used by viruses but not human cells. Human cells use a program written in DNA. Normally RNA and DNA messages are incompatible, but the virus wishes to use the T cell to reproduce itself. To do this it must get a message into the T cell's computer (nucleus) and change the instructions already encoded. To accomplish this, the HIV virus carries along with it an enzyme (called reverse transcriptase) that changes the program; in other words, the RNA message becomes a DNA message and this is inserted into the nucleus of the T cell. The T cell now has no choice but to turn its cellular factory over to the production of HIV. For every one virus that enters a T cell, a thousand identical copies will be made. As these new viruses are crowded inside the parasitised T cell, they start to burrow their way out of the cell and in so doing rupture and therefore kill the cell.

The HIV has attacked and killed its enemy but not before it has allowed it to survive long enough to produce new virus to go out and enslave even more T cells. These properties of the virus make it both fascinating and frightening and may allow it to slowly but surely kill every T 4 cell in our bodies.

One final feature about the envelope is worth understanding. Except for the previously mentioned probe, the remainder of the envelope constantly changes its structure. This is a trick well known to parasites such as the one that causes malaria. The technical name for this phenomenon is antigenic drift and the concept is straightforward enough. Cells of the immune system recognise a specific structure and call for help from other cells capable of attacking this particular three-dimensional structure. If the alarm goes out to attack the virus with the red coat but the virus changes into a blue coat before the army arrives, it escapes the melee. These biological attributes of the virus are worth detailing, for once people understand the challenge presented to us by this virus, they can understand why the progress of medical science towards a cure is not likely to be rapid. The immediate emphasis therefore must be placed on preventing HIV infection.

We have previously met viruses that have evolved to a point where they could at least temporarily damage part of the immune system. For instance, the Epstein-Barr virus (EBV) that causes 'mono' can damage B cells, but T cells will eventually kill off all the infected B cells and in that way destroy the virus. These are amateurs compared to the AIDS virus.

From the biological point of view, what is really significant about AIDS is the fact that a virus has learned how to cripple the immune system by killing off the single most crucial cell in our weaponry. A healthy human being has 200 billion to 300 billion T 4 cells circulating in the body but, enormous though that number is, the biological fact is that adults cannot make any more. By the time adulthood is reached, the thymus gland has retired.

Slowly but surely, the virus starts to decrease the number of T cells in the blood. From having 1000 or more T 4 cells in every tiny drop of blood in the body, there may gradually be absolutely none in a drop of blood as the AIDS virus does its work. Such a disaster does not occur overnight, but the disease and its long incubation period are best understood by considering that for many patients infected with the AIDS virus, some T 4 cells are lost with every tick of the clock. The day will inevitably come when there are simply not enough T 4 cells left to protect the body, and AIDS becomes recognisable.

We must now discuss infected blood. The blood of victims infected with the AIDS virus is just as infectious, if not more so, than the seminal fluid of such people. The blood of people suffering from an infection with the AIDS virus contains T 4 cells, T 4 cells contain virus and therefore the disease can be spread if blood containing infected T 4 cells enters a body.

Thus, soon after AIDS arrived and its association with sexual behaviour was noted, the same syndrome turned up in intravenous drug addicts, hemophiliacs and recipients of transfused infected blood.

My first patients with AIDS contracted as a result of an intravenous drug habit were a husband and wife.

Peter and Jo were not typical drug addicts; apparently they were both successful and happy. Peter wrote a nationally syndicated column telling people how to look after their house plants. His wife Jo was a psychiatric nurse, very much involved in her profession and working fulltime in an academic psychiatric institute. They were childless.

Jo had started using heroin while she was still at college. She remembers being quite scared of the whole drug scene during college and indeed it was not until her final year that she fell into an ever-more-common trap. One night after they had made love, her boyfriend told her that he found that heroin made the experience even more intensely pleasurable and urged her to share it with him. She allowed him to inject her with some heroin, which certainly had the effect he described.

For many months they shared heroin after lovemaking and insidiously addiction developed. Eventually, Jo broke the relationship with her boyfriend, but not her drug addiction. Shortly after the romance ended, Peter entered Jo's life and she introduced him to exactly the same pleasures and horrors.

At the time I first met them, their drug addiction was under some control. Because of the enormous costs involved in a daily heroin habit the couple had placed themselves on a regimen which consisted of daily maintenance therapy with methadone (a narcotic drug taken by mouth) which Jo would steal from the hospital where she worked. This kept them reasonably satisfied from Monday to Friday but on the weekends they splurged and went by themselves to a shooting gallery in New York. On Saturday mornings the couple would drive from their rural home in Connecticut into New York City and, in what they admit was a particularly seedy shooting gallery in one of the poorest parts of Brooklyn, they would buy their heroin.

They were aware of the infectious risks associated with drug addiction. Jo was treating a number of drug addicts and had seen how many had contracted hepatitis B infections because they shared needles with other drug addicts at the time that they 'shot up' their drugs. Syringes and needles are difficult to come by and are used time and time again by drug addicts, who make little attempt to clean them properly. Indeed, modern needles and syringes are meant to be disposable and it is not really possible to clean them adequately.

Jo and Peter avoided these problems by using sterile equipment whenever they injected drugs intravenously. Jo's hospital was the unwitting supplier of the equipment. They frequently took needles, syringes and a bottle of water for injection to the shooting gallery in Brooklyn, where they would buy their drug, suspend it in the sterile water and inject it immediately.

The couple were able to pinpoint with great accuracy the exact moment in which they met the AIDS virus. Only once Jo, who was responsible for bringing the equipment, thought she had put it in the car but had in fact left it behind on the dining-room table. As a result, when the couple arrived in Brooklyn, now quite desperate for their heroin, no safe equipment for injecting the drug was available to them. In their desperation they decided to gamble and use other people's needles and syringes.

The man from who they borrowed equipment was obliging but clearly emaciated and generally unwell. They knew him by his first name as they had seen him on a number of occasions in the gallery and they were later able to tell me that they discovered eighteen months later that he was in hospital desperately ill with this strange new disease called AIDS.

Jo and Peter suffered a severe flulike illness that hit them both approximately two weeks after their visit to the shooting gallery. For a week or so they had severe sweats, felt exhausted and even visited their local doctor, who understandably told them they had a flu that was going around and to rest up until it passed. The symptoms passed but the virus did not.

Not for a further year did any health problems descend on them. In the six months prior to seeing me, however, they had developed swollen glands, had lost weight, sweated frequently at night, suffered from attacks of stiffness in the hands on waking in the morning and had periodic rashes on the back and chest. Peter was more affected than Jo.

In the United States and many other countries, drug use is still a major factor in the continuing spread of the AIDS epidemic. As little as two drops of infected blood containing T 4 cells infected with the virus can deliver a fatal dose of the AIDS virus when injected into the bloodstream of another person. Experience has shown that it is much more difficult to modify the behaviour of drug addicts than it is, for example, to change the sexual customs of gay men.

You will now see why AIDS has become such a serious problem for patients who suffer from hemophilia. This group is suffering most severely from the AIDS epidemic, certainly suffering the most from the problems associated with contaminated blood. This group feel more bitterness and frustration than other victims of the disease. Hemophilia is a somewhat rare genetic condition that affects only males. The defective gene is carried by the mother who, although not affected, may pass it on to a son who will develop the disease. Most people know of bleeders, people who can bleed for hours, even days, if they suffer the slightest cut. Not all bleeders are hemophiliacs, but most are.

Almost as interesting as the immune system, and designed along similar lines, is our blood clotting system. When a blood vessel is cut or torn in a way that would allow blood to leak or even pour from the breach, an emergency of some proportion is signalled. All the blood circulates through major blood vessels every sixty seconds so it would be possible to exsanguinate remarkably quickly if a major vessel was opened.

The cells lining damaged blood vessels release chemicals that attract cells in the bloodstream called platelets. These cells are made in the bone marrow, and plugging leaks in blood vessels is their biological task. They do this every day for all of us because even if you bump your side on a table, tiny blood vessels would leak blood, causing a bruise, were it not for this mechanism. All of us injure ourselves constantly without even knowing it.

The platelets plug up the leak with their bodies but signal for stronger and more permanent repair work to be started immediately. In the bloodstream are twelve factors called, logically enough, blood clotting factors. These are activated in chain-gang fashion and when the end of the reaction is reached, a new wall of fibrin is built that can manage until the blood vessel grows its new wall.

Hemophiliacs lack one of the twelve factors; factor VIII. As a result, they cannot repair efficiently even the most minor breach in blood vessel walls. If they cannot make any factor VIII, they are in constant and terrible danger of bleeding to death. Some hemophiliacs can make some factor VIII so the disease has grades of severity.

Severe hemophiliacs have led miserable, boring lives until recent years. Either they were almost literally wrapped in cotton wool to protect them, or they battled on, but bled time and time again. Their joints suffered particularly because the joints are, of course, subjected to strains and bumps continuously, and small amounts of blood leaking into the joints would eventually destroy them, causing crippling arthritis.

Scientists discovered how to extract factor VIII from normal blood. Not only could the factor be extracted but it also could be concentrated and packaged so that bleeding could be rapidly controlled by an intravenous injection of the missing factor.

Producing commercial quantities of this factor required a lot of blood and it was soon realised that asking people to donate blood would not supply enough of the precious red stuff for this task. The volunteer pool was simply not big enough to maintain normal blood supplies and make enough blood available for factor VIII production. The commercial companies involved decided that they must buy the blood and so centers were set up where one could sell a unit of blood for cash.

From the outset it was realised that the 'sellers' would, to a large extent, be desperate people and that a number of drug addicts and the like would avail themselves of the ready cash. However, all donors were and are screened by physicians and all blood harvested was, and is, thoroughly checked for the hepatitis virus and every other known problem. The system worked well. The life of the hemophiliac was revolutionised.

Their tragedy, of course, is AIDS. Drug addicts and homesexuals infected with the virus lined up to sell their blood for factor VIII production. The collected blood pooled for commercial use became infected with the HIV virus that no one could detect at the time. Small amounts of the lethal virus were distributed in thousands of vials of factor VIII to the hemophiliacs of the world. On a per capita basis they are far and away the most affected and infected high-risk group. More than 70 per cent of the 12,000 hemophiliacs in the United States, for example, have been infected with the virus. Let me introduce you to one of the most remarkable.

Michael was thirty-two years old when I met him, seeking help for a severe cough and difficulty in breathing. He had a high fever and was clearly distressed but he had one of those irrepressible personalities which made him minimise his suffering. His fiancee, a nurse, was with him; their wedding was planned for a few months ahead. This remarkable hemophiliac had done something no one else afflicted with the disease had managed. From his earliest years, Michael was crazy about flying. Like so many little boys, he wanted to be the pilot of a big commercial jet; an impractical ambition for a hemophiliac but his was a fairly mild form of the disease and he ended up at the age of thirty-two as captain of a commercial airliner.

Throughout his life he had required factor VIII on only a few occasions and he had not received any for many years when he sprained his ankle one day in 1980. He went to his local hospital, concerned that this degree of trauma might lead to a dangerous amount of bleeding into his ankle joint. The ankle was strapped and his physician told him that, though it seemed all right, Michael should have some intravenous factor VIII 'just to be on the safe side'. Michael was doubtful, but eventually agreed. He received a bottle of contaminated factor VIII.

Michael had pneumonia when I first met him and was severely anemic. The pneumonia was the one that so frequently troubles victims of AIDS but the anemia puzzled us. Michael had not been bleeding and our investigations soon revealed that a nasty form of tuberculosis had invaded his bone marrow and was stopping him from producing blood.

For the next nine months, Michael struggled with the disease. He was very religious and his faith and courage kept him cheerful, even when he became covered with sores caused by a herpes infection. Amazingly, he died without bitterness.

How do children get AIDS? Like adults, they can contract the disease if they receive a transfusion of contaminated blood or blood products, but this is not the most common way they meet the virus.

Seth was only two when he first came to my clinic, the cute black child of a black mother and a smart but careless black father who is currently in the care of the government for two years.

Seth was 'failing to thrive'. He had big nodes in his neck and a big spleen, and he kept having one infection after another. It took us a few months in the early phase of the AIDS epidemic to work out what was amiss with Seth, but when the penny dropped we wanted to know how this two-year-old had contracted the disease.

We tested his mother and found that she had an early form of the infection. We tested the father (who was in prison) and he was perfectly well. His mother swore she was no drug addict and we believed her, nor had she had any blood transfusions. What Seth's mother had was a lover who was an intravenous drug addict. He was infected with the AIDS virus and had donated the virus to both mother and baby. She was pregnant when she met this man.

The AIDS virus can cross the placenta, moving from the mother's bloodstream to the baby's developing T cells. That is the way most children catch this disease.

Recently we have found that the virus is excreted in the breast milk of an infected mother and that a child suckling at the breast could be infected in this way. As was mentioned earlier, Nature has seen to it that T cells are in breast milk and we presume that the ingestion of infected T cells leads to the infection of the baby.

These cases illustrate how one can become infected with the AIDS virus. These are the only ways in which you can get infected. You cannot get it by accepting money from a gay man or washing your clothes in a laundromat frequented by gay men, nor from swimming pools, public toilets, cutlery, crockery, etc.

The tragedy of AIDS has been immeasurably compounded by people's ignorance of the disease, which has led to much unjustified fear and therefore an unjustified shunning of its victims. People have lost their jobs and their friends just for whispering that they were checked for AIDS. The role of the media in all this and even the inappropriate behaviour of some people in the medical profession deserves to be analysed and criticised.

Because of the slow evolution of the disease, we can recognise stages of the infection. Soon after infection, people are likely to feel well, with no signs of their disease on examination. Only education of high-risk groups will have them knocking on the door asking to be tested at this early stage.

Some people have some resistance to the infection, while others put up little in the way of a fight. A second stage can develop when patients have symptoms and signs. Swollen glands develop and profuse sweating at night, weight loss, stiffness in the joints and loss of libido and well-being are all common. Even these patients may, at least for many years, stay static, having apparently reached some form of compromise with the virus. Unfortunately most patients with constitutional symptoms will slip into the disease AIDS. Studies in the Western world have shown that 36 per cent of people initially infected with the virus have developed AIDS after seven years of follow-up. We have no crystal ball to tell us what percentage will eventually get AIDS but unfortunately the number has increased with each year of our experience.

By the time you read this, one feels confident that education will have significantly reduced the incidence of new cases. Fear of the disease will have abated among the general population (and, of course, among those who read this book).

Using the present leads and knowledge of the immune system scientists must come up with two strategies that can be used simultaneously before patients with AIDS can be cured. We need to restore T cell function to victims with the terminal form of the illness and simultaneously develop and administer drugs that will poison the virus and stop it from multi-plying.

In many countries, one agent, Retrovir, is being trialled. This drug shows considerable promise and is discussed further below. Using such a drug and a bone marrow transplant, at least one patient might have been cured of the disease. A man in America was fortunate enough to have an identical twin brother who was healthy. As we have discussed previously, normal bone marrow contains T cells. For most bone marrow transplant operations we are very anxious to eradicate those T cells. However, with an identical twin this is not necessary and indeed the T cells in the bone marrow were able to repopulate the body of the man, who would otherwise have died of AIDS. By using a drug to cripple the virus, these new T cells were able to take hold and eradicate the HIV. Very few people have identical twin brothers, but at least this case report had demonstrated to immunologists and biologists alike that the combined approach of improving T cell function (which may require a thymus transplant) and simultaneously using antiviral agents, a cure for AIDS may be developed.

The HIV virus has now been detected in 136 countries and many of the others haven't really looked diligently to see if they have the problem. The World Health Organisation considers 12 million people to be infected with the virus; 36 per cent of these will die in the next seven to eight years unless we have a major therapeutic breakthrough. Africa may have six million of its people infected; the USA has 1.5 million cases of infection. The human tragedy, the disruption of medical services and the financial burden of the epidemic, is nothing short of disastrous.

In 1990 in the USA more than 174,000 cases of AIDS will be admitted to hospital and half of those patients will die in that year. The care of these patients and the fight to prevent new infections will cost the United States billions of dollars over the next few years. The World Health Organisation has established in Geneva a huge and expensive taskforce to fight AIDS worldwide. From here they constantly remind us that AIDS is a global tragedy that will demand a response from all of us.

HIV infections continue to spread rapidly in Africa. Heterosexual transmission of the virus accounts for almost all cases, as this is a disease of sexually active young people. This fact allowed epidemiologists to rule out mosquitoes as a vector even before specific studies of the transmission of HIV by mosquitoes were performed. For transmission by mosquito, we would have needed a new breed that favored the blood of sexually active young Africans. In some cities of tropical Africa, 80 per cent of the population of child-bearing age are infected with the virus. When you consider that most African countries can afford only between seventeen and forty cents per capita per year on health services and that one HIV antibody test costs a minimum of $2, then it becomes immediately clear that we will all need to make a massive effort to supply technical and financial support to underdeveloped countries fighting HIV.

AIDS has now reached Asia with nearly 300 cases documented. Given the scanty attention paid to the virus in Asia to date, these figures are alarming. Many Asians believed, inaccurately, that they might be more immune to the effects of the HIV virus than other races. Geography, not genetics, protected Asia in the first few years of the epidemic. Of very great significance is the discovery that AIDS in Asia is spreading largely through heterosexual activity and that in countries like Indonesia, the Philippines and Malaysia, it is the genital health of women that may be the most important single determinant of the rate of the diseases spread.

The major issues and controversies

The AIDS epidemic has allowed many societies to see their weaknesses and strengths in the clearest of lights. Prejudice and ignorance, always bad bedfellows, have led to attitudes and decisions that have increased suffering and hindered the implementation of policies that would minimise the spread of the disease. On the other hand, many individuals and organisations have worked furiously, compassionately and intelligently to meet the challenge. As a result we have many controversies to deal with but many new facts to help with this task.

HIV antibody test

Seeking the fingerprints of the HIV virus in an individual by screening his blood for antibodies to the virus remains our best tool for following the flow of the epidemic, planning for future health services and helping, through early diagnosis, an infected individual. Despite all these worthwhile uses of antibody testing, screening programs remain controversial.

The test itself is no longer controversial; its strengths and weaknesses have been clearly defined. Eighty per cent of individuals infected with the HIV virus declare this to be the case by producing circulating antibodies to the virus in their blood two to three weeks after infection. Almost 100 per cent do so by three months after infection. A recent report from Finland of two individuals who did not develop antibodies for fifteen months after infection is of interest, but is so rare that it is not significant in the general context of testing and diagnosis. In any case, the Finnish data have been challenged by a number of scientists who feel that the problems they reported lay with the testing methods used rather than the patients' antibody system.

Antibody testing does have to deal with one obvious and unavoidable weakness: if someone has a negative antibody test, all that can be said is that, if that individual could not have been infected with the virus in the three months prior to the test, he or she is not infected with HIV. If they could have met the virus in that time period, they will need a second test after three months in which there has been no possible exposure. Then, and only then, can the all-clear signal be sounded. In the majority of studies any delay in sero-conversion is not a problem.

The handling of the results, not the performance of the tests, continues to produce controversy. HIV antibody screening is not just another test. A positive result tells an individual that he or she has a life-threatening infection. It may also abolish any quality their life may have because of the discrimination that may follow. Time and time again I have seen individuals who have shared the burden of knowing they are infected with HIV with a friend (a problem shared is a problem halved), immediately lose their friend.

Some families withdraw and even throw an HIV-infected member out into the street. Schools reject HIV-infected children. Recently a court in Florida, having reviewed the scientific evidence, ordered a school to educate three infected children on the school premises. The teachers and parents obeyed the order by buying, from their own money, a caravan and placing it in the far corner of the schoolyard, confining the three children to the caravan during school hours and calling for volunteers to teach these little 'lepers'.

If an individual is considering being tested in such a climate, he obviously weighs carefully the pros and cons of the exercise. If the test is negative he may be mightily relieved but if it is positive, can the information help him as an individual? If he is to risk discrimination he will not be interested in our desire to gather statistics on the speed at which the disease is spreading. If misguided governments have, as is unfortunately the case in a number of countries, introduced penalties with which to punish those people infected with the HIV virus who have sex with anyone without telling them of their infection, then voluntary screening for the HIV antibody seems even less appealing. A jealous lover could accuse one of all kinds of indiscretions. If, as is also the case in many places, laws have been passed which allow health officials to demand from doctors the names and address of individuals tested if they feel they need that information, individuals who contemplate being tested are further troubled.

Early diagnosis of HIV infection is helpful for a given patient. His battle with the HIV virus can be assisted and complications treated. But for the community, even more than for the individual, testing is essential and it is therefore necessary for all countries to work diligently to remove impediments to voluntary screening programs.

Why such widespread discrimination continues is worth examining, indeed researching. Given the irrefutable evidence that you can catch the HIV from another only if his or her blood or sexual secretions enter your body, why is there so much fear that leads to rejection? Prejudice against homosexual men is part of the problem. At a meeting of mortuary attendants who had refused to assist with autopsies on patients dying from AIDS, I was asked, 'Why should we put ourselves at risk by cutting up a dead poofter?' No amount of explaining the facts, including the obvious one that not all AIDS victims are gay, had any effect on these men.

Recently a patient of mine in the terminal phases of his struggle with AIDS, decided he would like one final weekend in his attractive apartment by the sea. A heterosexual and single man of fifty years, he had been infected by sexual intercourse with a prostitute. All his life he had been involved with the surf lifesaving movement and was a champion swimmer and instructor. His club was his life. One of his young prodigies who had been asked to get some food into the apartment for this last weekend at home, called me to ask if Bill was well enough to enjoy a surprise. Twenty of the lads from the surf lifesaving association wanted to be there when he arrived home to pay their respects, show their appreciation of his help in years gone by and sadly to say goodbye. It was well known that Bill was dying. Bill had not hidden this fact from his friends, but had chosen to tell them that he was dying from cancer.

I thought the surprise party was a wonderful idea. An ambulance was ordered to take Bill home on a Saturday afternoon for the weekend.

On Sunday morning while on a ward round of my patients in the AIDS unit, I passed Bill's room. To my surprise, he was in his bed sobbing quietly. Enquiries soon revealed how the surprise party had gone sadly astray.

The ambulance men who picked up Bill from our AIDS unit, despite the protestations of the patient and staff, wore space suits. They were covered from head to feet and wore thick yellow kitchen gloves. Bill was amazed but did not know what was waiting for him at his home and therefore resigned himself to their stupidity and his embarrassment. When the gathering awaiting Bill saw him being carried into his apartment by these weirdly dressed ambulance men, surprise gave way to consternation. The true cause of Bill's illness was revealed to his friends and to his gaping neighbours.

There was no party. All but one of our well-meaning but ignorant young men vanished and a distraught Bill, who had not wanted his friends to know of his AIDS, let alone feel their rejection, came back to hospital to die in misery two days later.

I was furious with the ambulance officers who had not followed the guidelines laid down and accepted by their organisation for the transfer of AIDS patients. When I confronted the ambulance officers involved, one of them defended his actions with a defiant 'you guys don't know as much as you think you know'.

This was a telling phrase, typical of a new attitude among many to medical science and the doctors that practise it. We constantly see intelligent people, who could not have escaped information on the lack of infectivity of AIDS from social intercourse, acting unintelligently: magistrates who refuse to have HIV-infected individuals in their courtrooms, policemen who demand danger money for arresting an HIV-infected prostitute, airline personnel who won't have such people in their planes, etc.

The changing attitudes of many to orthodox science and doctors may be attributed, no doubt, to many different factors. With a breakthrough behind us that saw vaccines and antibiotics developed to wipe out so much of the suffering of mankind, we find ourselves in a period when the tough problems remain tough and yield their secrets reluctantly. We need breakthroughs in cancer, heart disease and even ageing to win back many who expected the flow of medical miracles to continue.

Physicians must assume some of the blame. Too many of them, in these difficult economic times, practise turnstile medicine, dispensing good drugs for poor reasons as they fail to give the patient sufficient time to explore exactly what is and what is not wrong with them. Sadly there are many of us teachers of medicine who feel the standard of medical practice in the Western world is falling despite more practical knowledge being available than ever before.

In fact, the rapidity with which sound, useful and complex knowledge about the HIV virus and its ravages has accumulated is a triumph of modern medicine. We have much to learn about the HIV virus, of course, but there will be no retreating from the established fact that only when HIV-infected secretions—blood and occasionally breast milk— enter one's body, is there any chance of becoming infected.

The world's scientific community has accepted a new classification system for HIV infection that will ensure uniformity in data collection. Antibody testing is a vital part of that classification system. Patients with HIV infection are now placed in one of four groups. Group I patients are those who have only recently been infected and are experiencing the flulike illness that is so unexceptional in most cases that it is not even remembered. This illness coincides with the appearance in the bloodstream of antibodies to HIV. Group II contains the majority of patients infected with HIV. They are totally well, infected, and most importantly, infectious. Group III contains individuals who have developed swollen lymph glands and some of the constitutional symptoms associated with an HIV infection; night sweats, weight loss, etc. Group IV contains those patients with any of the serious consequences that follow HIV infection including the most severe complication of all, AIDS.

Other complications include Kaposi's sarcoma and the neurological complications of the HIV invasion of the brain. This latter increasingly recognised complication can so rapidly destroy brain tissue that an intelligent, fully functional human can be reduced to senile dementia in just six weeks.

Who should be tested?

- Anyone who is worried for any reason. Often a test is needed to dispel unwarranted fears that will not evaporate, even with expert counselling.
- All gay men who have been sexually active in the last years.
- All hemophiliacs who have received factor VIII.
- Everyone who had a transfusion of blood or blood products (plasma, platelets, etc.) between 1978 and May of 1985 when antibody testing of all blood donors was introduced. Some countries still do not test blood donors and in such countries the risk of acquiring HIV from a transfusion remains.
- Individuals who have had sex (especially anal sex) with a prostitute, particularly in Africa or in Asia.
- All male and female prostitutes.
- All intravenous drug users who have ever shared a needle or syringe.

- All sexual partners of intravenous drug users.
- All children born to HIV-infected mothers.
- All donors for sperm banks.
- All donors of organs for transplantations.
- All blood donors.
- All prisoners.
- All members of the armed forces.
- All diplomatic personnel sent to countries where AIDS is a major problem and the blood supply is not screened.

In many societies where HIV infection is a major problem, women planning pregnancy should be tested, as should immigrants moving from those countries to any others. Couples in an evolving relationship will much more commonly seek reassurance from each other that their previous sexual experiences have not exposed them to HIV. This will be necessary before sexual intimacy can safely take its place within that relationship. Unromantic? Yes. Necessary? In many places, definitely. The advice will hold for many more cities and countries in the not-too-distant future, unless we halt the spread of this disease.

Because of continuing discrimination problems, no one should have the HIV antibody test without the advantage of prior counselling about the consequences of a positive result. Similarly, immediate counselling must be available to those whose tests turn out to be positive. Pretest counselling should include a discussion of the discrimination that abounds, the necessity of keeping the news of a positive result to a very limited number of people, the inability of HIV-positive individuals to get life assurance, the fact that being HIV positive is not synonymous with having AIDS, etc.

Antigen testing

One technical problem associated with antibody testing will be solved by antigen tests. None of the discrimination problems will disappear, however. By antigen testing is meant the detection of the virus itself, rather than antibody to the virus. Antigen testing is rapidly improving as more and more sensitive techniques are forwarded that allow us to search a patient's blood for minute amounts of the proteins that make up both the coat and the core of the virus. These proteins can be detected within twenty-four hours of infection but the amount present in the blood then decreases through considerable time before returning in full force. Techniques for antigen testing have to be very sensitive to ensure that false negatives are not reported. At this writing we are just about there. Antigen testing, in combination with antibody testing, will be routine within a year.

Antigen testing will be invaluable in helping us diagnose HIV infections in the newborn babies of infected mothers. All these infants have antibodies against HIV in their blood but it may be antibody produced by the mother, not by the baby. Only when all the maternal antibody disappears and is replaced by the baby's own gammaglobulin (about the age of one), can a diagnosis of HIV infection be made by antibody screening. Antigen testing will solve that problem. Antigen testing will also eliminate the vulnerability that troubles blood banks. Theoretically, donors who have been infected within three months of giving blood could nevertheless have a positive antibody test. While in practice this has not been a problem, the advantages of the antigen tests are obvious.

Heterosexual AIDS

There is a frightening complacency among many heterosexual individuals about the potential of the AIDS epidemic to affect them. Why is it so difficult to get an appropriate tone into the debate about the risk of HIV transmission by heterosexual activity? On the one hand we have insufficiently informed individuals declaring authoritatively that heterosexuals having vaginal intercourse have nothing to fear from the HIV virus. They claim that calling for a modification of sexual behavior among heterosexuals can come only from moralists or homosexuals who wish to have the heterosexual community sexually shackled like themselves. At the other extreme, we have statements from individuals who see AIDS as a punishment for sin and predict that soon the heterosexual community will be afflicted by a massive plague that will indeed sweep away the sexually promiscuous.

As is so often the case in hotly debated issues, the truth is very much in the middle. Here are the facts. You can decide for yourself.

Women having anal sex in which HIV-infected seminal fluid or even the secretions that emerge from the penis prior to ejaculation enter their rectum, face the same risk experienced by a gay male in a similar situation. While it is entirely possible that one such episode could lead to a fatal infection, statistical analysis of the available data tells us that one's chance of becoming infected after ten to fifty such episodes with an infected male is about 48 per cent. Is trauma necessary? I don't think so, but there is no doubt that bleeding or the tearing of mucous membranes would increase the risk, as would any anal or rectal sore. Many men and women who regularly engage in anal sex are able to dilate their anal sphincter readily and not be traumatised by an erect penis. Recent studies in the USA show that 10 per cent of women regularly engage in anal sex for pleasure; 25 per cent do so occasionally. On these figures, more women have anal sex in the USA than men.

What are the risks for a woman who has only vaginal intercourse with an infected man? Some variables are to be considered here. The infectiousness of a man's sexual secretions increase with time; it becomes even more dangerous as his T-cell count begins to fall. As the years of the epidemic pass, we have seen a big increase in the number of infected wives married to hemophiliacs or men themselves infected by a blood transfusion. Thus it is important for women to realise that some infected men are far more dangerous than others. One African man who visited Europe and had only vaginal sex with sixteen European women infected nine of them.

As is the case with anal sex, vaginal sex can result in infection after only one episode. I care for a number of patients who have had this experience. However, statistics tell us that repeated exposure is usually necessary. To try and quantify the risk, a review of the world's literature and my own experience would suggest that a woman who has vaginal intercourse with an infected man between ten and fifty times has a 17 to 33 per cent chance (mean 26 per cent chance) of being infected. These statistics can be dangerous.

A recent report on a wire service told women all around the world the good news from one study. Sixty-six per cent of the wives or regular lovers of HIV-infected men who had in fact being living with these men for a year were not themselves infected with HIV at the end of that period. The virus is not so bad after all!

Surely such a report should have contained a completely different emphasis. What a tragedy it is that 34 per cent of the lovers of HIV-infected men have themselves become infected with the deadly virus. The English have a pithy advertisement on billboards in which an elegant young woman looks you in the eye and says, 'I like sex, but I am not prepared to die for it.'

The other variable that must be re-emphasised is the genital health of women. While the infection of women during artificial insemination tells us that neither trauma nor an obvious break of the vaginal lining is necessary for infection, strong data indicate that women with genital ulcers, cervical erosions, a previous history of gynecological surgery or sexually transmitted diseases are significantly more vulnerable. Genital problems are very frequently found in underdeveloped countries but they are anything but uncommon in Western society. Without regular inspection of the genital tract, many women could be unaware of the existence of some of these problems, for symptoms may be minimal.

What about oral sex? If a woman allows male (or female) sexual secretions to enter her mouth or swallows such secretions, can she be infected? Here the data are circumstantial. We know that HIV can infect babies fed infected breast milk. We know that infected blood, taken inadvertently into the mouth of health professionals, has resulted in their infection and we have one case report where a lesbian was infected by taking infected secretions from her female lover into her mouth. The risk from oral sex we believe is minimal but not insignificant; it is, after all, a deadly virus of which we speak.

Infection of heterosexual men

A man having anal sex with an infected woman faces the same risks he would experience if his partner were an infected male. His chances of being infected from vaginal intercourse alone can be looked at statistically. With ten to fifty episodes of vaginal intercourse with an HIV-infected woman, he faces a 12 to 15 per cent chance of becoming infected. Again, a number of variable factors greatly change the risk for a given individual. Abrasions, cuts or ulcers on the penis increase the risk considerably but it should be emphasised that macroscopic (as opposed to microscopic) breaks in the skin of the penis are not necessary for infection. It is quite possible that the sexual secretions of a woman could contain so much virus that some HIV could enter the body through the urethra (the opening in the penis).

Recently sixteen healthy English engineers spent six months in Africa on a construction job for their company. Fifteen of them returned to Britain infected with HIV contracted by vaginal sex with African prostitutes. In underdeveloped countries the risk for men appears to be greater; 55 per cent of male partners of HIV-infected women in Haiti have themselves been infected.

The cervical and vaginal secretions of HIV-infected women contain virus and virus-infected T cells episodically. Virus can be recovered from vaginal secretions at a time it cannot be recovered from blood. Vaginal virus is not related to the menstrual cycle and does not represent a spillover from blood. A woman, however, may be more infectious and more vulnerable to infection during her period.

The HIV virus will never spread through the heterosexual community in the West at the speed with which it devastated the gay community. Reassuring articles are written because of this, often quoting the fact that in the USA only 3 to 6 per cent of the known cases of HIV infection have occurred in heterosexual men and women whose only risk factor was sex with a carrier. But imagine that you picked up the paper one morning to find a headline: 'Ninety thousand heterosexual Americans infected with a deadly virus spread by sexual intercourse'. That is the reality in the USA and the Center for Disease Control tells us that the doubling rate for new heterosexual cases is ten months. Three per cent does not sound much but it certainly represents a lot of suffering when you realise that 1.5 million Americans are infected.

Surely we need to make every effort to stop this virus from spreading through the heterosexual community. Unless sexual behaviour is modi-fied, it will spread relatively slowly but inexorably into this community and we should in no way be complacent about the matter. Studies in Western societies have revealed very similar data. Thirty to thirty-five per cent of young people in the fifteen to twenty-seven age bracket regularly engage in activities that will facilitate the spread of this disease.

Condoms

The promotion of condoms as a useful weapon in the fight against AIDS has been controversial everywhere. The scientific facts are clear. The HIV cannot pass through an intact condom. Provided a condom is used throughout the entire act of intercourse, does not break, and none of its contents are allowed to spill during withdrawal of the penis from the vagina or anus, the risk of HIV transmission in either direction is minimal. The problem is that years of experience in the use of condoms for contraceptive purposes tells us that a 5 to 10 per cent problem rate is to be expected. Tearing of the condom accounts for only 1 per cent of the problem and this risk is highest with anal intercourse. The major problem has been, and remains, user error.

There is a lot of resistance to the use of condoms, mainly by men, and unless the sheathing of the erect penis is done as part of sexual foreplay, there is often nothing to put a condom on. It takes practice. Women in most Western societies will have to insist on condoms and indeed carry them in their purse, given the attitudes of males towards this precaution-ary move. Numerous studies have shown that men will wear condoms if asked to do so, but are much less likely to suggest their use than women. There is reasonable scientific evidence to suggest that condoms containing the spermicide antiviral agent nonoxynolnine provides somewhat better protection that condoms without this agent.

The real controversy is confronted when health authorities try and promote the use of condoms. Some claim that such promotions will increase sexual activity among the young; there is no evidence for this, however. Others object to discussion of the subject on television and would never accept the type of demonstrations shown in Scandinavia and the United Kingdom in which a model of an erect penis was used for demonstrating the correct technique for using condoms.

Societies can be hypocritical in this regard. Recently I was waiting in a television studio to discuss the abandoning of effective television adver-tising of condoms on the grounds of public disquiet. In the studio where I was waiting I saw on the monitor, in glorious color, a movie about a man living in a Mediterranean villa with two women he loved and who also loved him. As the three of them frolicked by his beautiful pool in the altogether, the phones in the television studio were quite silent. The television interviewer and I looked at each other and laughed as the irony struck us both simultaneously.

The churches are struggling with the theology of condom usage as an anti-AIDS measure. If you use a condom to protect yourself from the AIDS virus and at the same time this prevents conception, can a married hemophiliac still have intercourse with his wife? Would a young teenage girl who has no intention of having intercourse with anyone be placed in the path of sin if she carried some condoms in her purse? While many of us are not troubled by such questions, they are important for thousands or indeed millions who look for guidance on this matter to church authorities.

Sex and AIDS education in schools

Many societies are having difficulty accepting the advice from most health authorities that children from the age of twelve years up need to be told about AIDS in language appropriate for their age but nevertheless explicit. School systems are not used to being called upon to assist in health emergencies. Many school systems in Europe and the United States responded rapidly, most have not and survey after survey tells us that children are still confused. In the western suburbs of Sydney, Australia, recently, an investigator seeking answers to an alarming increase in IV Amphetamine, used among teenagers, asked them, among other things, if they were not concerned about developing AIDS with all the needle sharing going on. 'Hell, no', was the answer. 'We're not gay.'

Aids and IV drug use

Most people who use IV drugs and share needles are not addicts but recreational users. Both groups share an equal risk of being infected with HIV. In many parts of the USA the sharing of needles has become the major method for HIV transmission. New Jersey is the best (worst?) example. On Manhattan island, 275,000 IV drug users are infected and health authorities have already decided to ignore them as they put all their energies into preventing new cases.

What can be done with the IV-drug-using population? Some can be educated and change, according to a recent report from San Francisco. Some can be taught to rinse their syringes and needles with household bleach before passing the equipment on to the next user. Some can be diverted from their IV use by accelerated acceptance into a well-run methadone program in which tablets are substituted for the IV drug. Perhaps the best but most controversial step is issuing free needles and syringes to drug users on an exchange basis. In Amsterdam, where the pilot program was conducted, 80 per cent of the needles and syringes were returned to the distributors. For many, however, the thought that we are giving sterile syringes and needles to people whom we desperately want to stop using drugs is distressing. Recently, in advocating acceptance of such a program to a group of clergymen who certainly looked doubtful, I used an 'ends justify the means' approach. An archbishop jumped up and gently rebuked me for suggesting this philosophy and emphasised the difference between 'the end justifies the means' and the lesser of two evils. He told us a story about St Thomas Aquinas and his efforts to establish brothels, not because he was in favour of prostitution, but because he could not stand to see the robberies and murders accociated with uncontrolled street prostitution. The archbishop won the day for me, I believe.

All authorities agree that in Western society HIV drug users are largely responsible for introducing the virus into the heterosexual community. It is an interesting fact that most of the female sexual partners of male IV drug users in the USA do not themselves use drugs. When the greatest of social ills is mixed with the greatest of social diseases, a disaster cocktail results.

Retrovir (AZT)

Recently a most exciting advance in the therapy of HIV infection has produced an ethical dilemma for governments and society. The British pharmaceutical giant Burroughs Wellcome developed a drug that markedly reduces the rate at which the AIDS virus can multiply. The drug is a DNA chain terminator. As the virus instructs T cells to cement together the building blocks that will construct a new AIDS virus, the drug binds to one of the blocks, preventing the next piece of the virus being correctly aligned. Given to patients in group III, that is, patients losing their battle with the virus but who have not yet developed AIDS, the drug can improve health and add between one and two years of quality life to 60 per cent of patients. It doesn't cure and it is less useful to patients with AIDS than to those with a less serious complication of HIV infection. Most patients with AIDS are young and our approach is based on the hope that a major curative breakthrough is around the corner. Retrovir is valuable for keeping patients as well as possible for as long as possible.

It is a very significant advance; the problem is one of expense. The drug costs about $US8000 per year per patient and it doesn't cure them. Many cannot afford the drug as they have lost their jobs and are heavily burdened with medical bills. In the USA only the wealthy and those helped by family or friends can afford it. In countries with a national health scheme governments are balking at the bill, especially as scientific evidence accumulates suggesting that we should give AZT to people in group II, i.e., the infected, infectious, but well patient. It may help them fight their HIV infection and we already know it reduces their risk of infecting a sexual partner. In a number of countries governments have said, 'No more'. A quota system has been introduced and after the quota has been supplied, no more government money will be available for the drug.

This has sparked a debate which must catch fire and spread. It is up to all of us in society to decide how many of the technical advances that are now or soon will be available to prolong an individual's life we can or will afford. From AZT to artificial hearts, the debate must lead to a societal discussion about the priorities we place on an individual's life. Certainly those of us who have to look into the eyes of a patient infected with the AIDS virus and tell them that they are a week too late for getting help from AZT, feel that no Western society has spent enough on this drug at this time. We all, however, realise there must be a limit. That limit cannot be set by doctors. For forty cents per week per patient, we could eliminate malaria, but we won't spend the money. Issues such as AIDS may force us to come to grips with decisions about affording what is possible but very expensive. Can a city build a new opera house while thousands of young people cannot be given a life-preserving drug? I suspect so.

The blood supply

Because most individuals infected with the HIV virus remain well for years, many infected people donated or sold blood to the Red Cross or commercial blood banks prior to May of 1985. Donated blood is more often than not split between two recipients; the red cells may be given to one patient and the plasma to another. Thousands of patients around the world were infected in this manner, when 100 per cent of people given an infected blood transfusion were themselves infected.

Vicious rumours circulated on a number of continents that gay men, infected with the HIV virus, deliberately gave blood to blood banks to ensure that the heterosexual community also became infected. There is no evidence to support such a claim anywhere in the world.

In May of 1985 most Western blood banks began the labor-intensive and expensive but obviously essential job of screening all blood donated for the presence of antibody to HIV. Well before this time they had introduced measures to deter individuals belonging to high-risk groups from donating blood. Written information was given to prospective donors explaining explicitly just who should not give. Combining anti-body testing with the completion of a detailed questionnaire, blood banks have virtually abolished the risk of contracting HIV from blood or a blood product. When antigen testing is available, the tiny risk that some pathological personality infected within a few weeks of donation will be able to lie his or her way through a questionnaire and escape detection by antibody screening will disappear. A number of problems remain, however.

In many countries hundreds, indeed thousands, of people infected by contaminated blood are unaware of their infection. This is bad news for them and of course means that their sexual partners are at risk. In the United States only 3000 of the 12,000 thought to have been infected in this manner have so far been found. For this reason many countries that can afford the gesture are asking patients who received blood or blood products during their country's vulnerable period (1978–1985 in the USA) to have an HIV antibody test. It is difficult to conduct such a look-back program without causing panic and rekindling fear about the blood supply today. In Sydney, Australia, 275,000 people will need to be screened in the attempt to find 400 infected recipients.

A further problem of considerable significance for travellers needs discussing. Many countries are not screening blood donors. Most cannot afford it (Africa, the Philippines, Indonesia and others) while some are remarkably tardy in introducing these measures. By the time you read this, one hopes that the situation will have changed, but travellers should know if a country that they plan to visit has a safe blood supply. This information is available from most airlines.

The lack of universal testing sees many diplomatic services demanding that all their personnel are HIV-tested before being dispatched to foreign posts. In this way they are able to rely on each other as a source of blood should this be necessary. Such reasoning lies behind the decision of many countries to test all personnel in the armed forces. In the latter case the realisation that HIV infection of the brain can alter the appropriateness of decisionmaking before the major complications of HIV infection are manifest has added impetus to the screening program.

The AIDS epidemic has seen the establishment of a number of private blood banks that will store your own blood for you in case you ever need small amounts close to home. This is a reasonable idea, though expensive. Of course such banks will not be able to help you if major trauma demands immediate transfusion or if your problems develop far from home. For this reason, it is important for all to realise that the blood supplied by banks that question their donors and screen their blood can now be considered perfectly safe.

Mosquitoes

Many find difficulty in believing that mosquitoes don't spread the HIV. They *don't*, and we now know why they can't. Careful scientific analysis of mosquitoes deliberately allowed to feed on HIV-infected blood has taught us that there is not sufficient blood left on the biting parts of the mosquito after a feed to have enough infected T cells pass on HIV to the mosquito's next victim. In addition, the virus passing into the mosquito's stomach cannot multiply and infect the mosquito. In fact, the virus is killed. Without replication the virus cannot be concentrated in the mosquito's salivary glands, a necessary step for the transmission of organisms when biting. Those diseases that mosquitoes do spread involve parasites or viruses that have adapted their lifestyle to enable them to survive and in some cases thrive inside the mosquito. We are indeed fortunate that in its modelling the HIV neglected the adaptation steps needed to use mosquitoes.

There are numerous other AIDS-related issues that we cannot discuss here but that are of great importance. Human life assurance policies for HIV-infected people and those in high-risk groups, the control of the spread of HIV in jails where intravenous drug use and 'institutional sex' is so common, intelligent policies for the schooling of HIV-infected children, the expansion of community services to handle the death of so many young people and the acceptance by government of their global responsibilities are but a few of the urgent issues needing resolution.

The HIV virus is presenting us with many serious challenges. His-torians will be able to tell much about us (if the HIV doesn't win) in their documentation of whether we were intelligent enough to eradicate a virus that could be beaten without a drug or a vaccine by simply modifying dangerous behaviour. As there are no signs that we have evolved to the point where we can accept that challenge, let us double our efforts to find a cure. At least five people have died of AIDS while you were reading this chapter, and fifty more have been infected with the virus.

PART IV WHERE ARE THE GENERALS?

7 | Understanding allergies

I N 1905, Austrian scientist Clemens Von Pirquet was involved in the research work that gave the world the term 'allergy' and pushed back the frontiers of the infant science of immunology. His work culminated in a huge manuscript which he published in an American medical journal in 1911. Sandwiched between an article on the hazards to women's health if they wore corsets too tightly, and the hazards of cross-infection in poorly ventilated trains was his eighty-five-page account entitled 'Allergy'.

To understand the significance of Von Pirquet's work, we need to spend a little time setting the scientific scene. It was known by the turn of the century that immunological protection (i.e., the reason why one does not get the same infection twice, etc.) was related to the appearance of chemicals in the blood of a person who has recovered from an initial infection. These chemicals were called 'antibodies'. There was no knowledge of the thymus gland's role in any of this, no knowledge of T cells; the concept of cells specifically attacking tissue invaders was forty years away.

Among infectious diseases in Europe, none was more devastating than tuberculosis, a killer with no respect for age. From the organisms that caused this disease Von Pirquet had isolated and extracted a protein that was very useful. It was harmless, as it was not infectious, but when injected into the skin of people one of two things would happen. Either no reaction would be noted or, slowly over forty-eight hours, a red itchy lump would appear at the injection site: a tuberculosis reaction. This latter was very important, for it meant that the bacteria that caused TB had been or were still in the body, and the immune system had responded or was responding. Patients with suspected TB but negative skin tests would have another cause for their problem.

Today, we can envisage the protein extract from the bacteria being recognised by T cells in the skin, and the alarm being sounded. Defense mechanisms are rushed in to do battle and if one has had previous experience with these organisms, one's defenses are so efficient that at the end of forty-eight hours a massive attack is under way and clearly visible. All Von Pirquet knew for certain was that a positive reaction meant that at some time the patient had come in contact with the organisms that caused tuberculosis.

In his experiments designed to learn more about this reaction, Von Pirquet used guinea pigs and another protein that was easier to come by—albumen—the protein in the white of the ordinary egg. If his theory about the tuberculosis reaction was correct, it would be necessary only to immunise or sensitise an animal with any protein and the telltale skin reaction would be checked. Injecting egg albumen into the skin of a sensitised guinea pig would produce the same reaction seen when the extract from the organisms that caused TB were injected into a patient with that disease.

What Von Pirquet found, however, was not what he expected. When he injected the egg material into the skin of the guinea pig, he noted an *immediate* reaction. Within minutes, sometimes within seconds, a red reaction occurred at the injection site. Clearly, this was quite different from the reaction that took forty-eight hours to develop with his TB extract.

Further research showed that this immediate reaction was no predictor of immunity and, in fact, could be dangerous. Sometimes, when Von Pirquet and other scientists interested in the same phenomena injected certain proteins such as egg albumen into the skin of immunised animals, not only would they get an immediate reaction, but they might also become acutely ill. Some of the animals would start to wheeze, gasp for breath and then die before the alarmed eyes of the scientists.

In his 1911 paper, Von Pirquet summarised all his work on the subject and formulated the following. Clearly, immunising an animal (even the human one) altered the energy level of the immune system's response to the material. A vigorous response characterises the sensitised individual. This altered state of immunological energy he called 'allergy', a word he compiled from two Greek words, *allos* meaning altered and *ergeai* meaning energy. Von Pirquet subdivided allergy into two forms, useful and useless. An immediate reaction to whatever you had been sensitised to was a useless, perhaps even dangerous, form of allergy. On the other hand, the delayed reaction was very useful.

Since 1911, the strict definition of the term 'allergy' as described by the coiner of the word has been modified. In most quarters, the word 'allergy' has become restricted to that useless but potentially dangerous form of immunity known more correctly as immediate hypersensitivity. Tuberculosis-type reactions are known as delayed hypersensitivity.

The fascinating story of Von Pirquet contains many other episodes of original discovery ranging from his observations on the medically beneficial effects of sunlight to important new knowledge about nutrition.

Von Pirquet had a reputation for not suffering fools gladly (he was a terrifyingly autocratic figure in his hospital) and a wife whom everyone thought was all wrong for him. She was not his mental or social equal. She was fat, lazy, unreasonably demanding and spoilt. Somehow, however, she had him where she wanted him; she often called him at his hospital and, despite a pressing conference or urgent experiment, he ran home to do her bidding. It was the strangest of relationships.

At the height of his fame, whilst still very productive, Von Pirquet went home from work one evening, made some efficient arrangements for his planned absence from the hospital and had a pleasant dinner with his wife featuring a good bottle of wine. He and his wife then moved out of this world via a couple of cyanide capsules. The world was so imperfect and so resistant to change that he and his wife had had enough.

And so we come to our examination of this important subject of 'allergy', an area of immunology that is shared by the best and worst scientists in our field, by some well meaning but misguided non-medical healers and those opportunistic charlatans who can make fortunes from the suffering of others.

The unpleasant effects induced by immediate hypersensitivity reactions are suffered by seventeen to twenty-four per cent of humans. Whether this reaction is triggered by pollen in our nose or airways, crayfish in our intestinal tract or a dose of penicillin in our buttocks, the mechanisms are identical to those noted by Von Pirquet when injecting egg protein into his guinea pigs.

We must begin by describing the mechanisms that cause immediate hypersensitivity reactions. For a long time we have known that the cause was circulating around in the body and was therefore likely to be an antibody. We owe that discovery to Drs Prausnitz and Kustner, members of that inquisitive German school of investigation that dominated medicine during the first years of this century.

These two scientists illustrated again what Louis Pasteur meant when he said that luck favors the prepared mind. Prausnitz and Kustner went out to dinner together one night. Kustner ordered fish, enjoyed it very much and then had a violent reaction to the meal. He developed itchy hives on his skin and wheezing as his bronchial tree suddenly spasmed and produced an acute attack of asthma. Clearly, Kustner had developed an 'allergy' to fish. This is a useless sort of immune response but obviously clinically important; people do die during allergic

HYPERSENSITIVITY

DELAYED HYPERSENSITIVITY

ANTIGEN
Dust
Pollens
Moulds
Food etc.

B CELL
recognises
ANTIGEN
and produces
IgE

IgE

IgE
plus
ANTIGEN
produces
immediate
explosion

HISTAMINE LIKE
CHEMICALS

Blood vessels
swell

Airways
narrow

Fluid leaks
out

Difficult
breathing

HIVES

ASTHMA

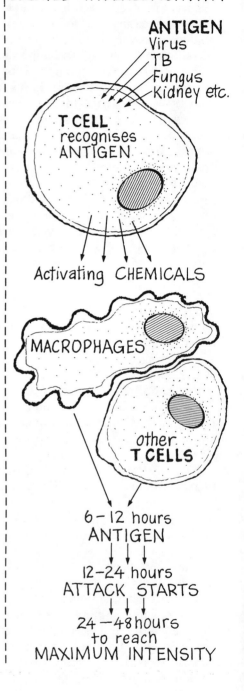

ANTIGEN
Virus
TB
Fungus
Kidney etc.

T CELL
recognises
ANTIGEN

Activating CHEMICALS

MACROPHAGES

other
T CELLS

6 – 12 hours
ANTIGEN

12 – 24 hours
ATTACK STARTS

24 – 48 hours
to reach
MAXIMUM INTENSITY

reactions of this type.

The two friends discussed the incident after Kustner had recovered and decided that one of their pet theories was ready for testing. If certain antibodies in the blood were responsible for allergic reactions to such things as fish, tomatoes, nuts and chocolates, etc., could one expect that an injection of serum obtained from an allergic individual into the body of one who is not allergic to a particular substance (eg, fish) would alter the state of immunological energy within the recipient, who would consequently acquire passively the allergic state of the donor?

Kustner's blood was taken, and the serum (the blood minus the cells contained in the blood) was injected under the skin on Prauznitz' arm. With that accomplished without ill effect, Kustner proceeded to the big test. What would happen if a little fish extract was injected into the skin where the serum had been placed?

A violent local allergic reaction occurred immediately. The scientists, in an unconventional but convincing manner, demonstrated that this allergic reaction was caused by something that circulated within the blood, presumably an antibody. That antibody we now call IgE: E for 'emergency' if you like.

Now, as was emphasised in the description of the immune system, there is nothing abnormal about manufacturing and secreting IgE. How *much* one makes is the important point here.

When you scratch your hand while pruning the roses and some bacteria get into the wound, a local battle must be fought if the defense system is to sterilise the wound and to allow healing to occur. Cells and antibodies needed for the job must be delivered to the infected scratch site via the blood flowing through the nearest blood vessel. It would clearly be an advantage if one could increase the blood supply adjacent to the scratch site. If tiny blood vessels in the skin around the scratch would only dilate; more blood could flow into the wound area.

After dilation the pores in the blood vessels, through which cells must escape if they are to enter the tissues, would be nicely stretched open. Blood vessels have circular, muscular coats wrapped around them. When the muscles contract less blood flows through the vessel; when the muscles relax, the opposite it true. The body can thus take more or less blood to a specific area as conditions warrant. Certain chemicals make the blood vessels relax, while others cause them to open up or dilate. Of the many chemicals that can be involved in such a reaction, the best known one is histamine.

Nature has designed a series of little chemical mines, i.e., cells full of different sorts of chemicals that can be exploded in the tissues when needed. Such cells are called mast cells and they are liberally scattered throughout our tissues.

To release these chemicals, IgE is needed. The mast cells which are full of chemicals such as histamine have a membrane that can bind IgE. A physical moiety on the cells' outer wall is complementary to a section of the tail of the IgE molecule. Once IgE binds to the mast cells, the latter are said to be 'armed'. All that is needed is something that can bind to the front end of the IgE which projects 'out', that is, away from the cells' membrane, and the explosive reaction will have occurred.

Once antigen and antibody combine, the mast cell explodes and releases the chemical it contains. By producing IgE very early in an immune response, Nature has supplied us with a 'gatekeeper' for blood vessels. By harnessing the chemicals in mast cells we can deliberately dilate blood vessels in areas under attack and unleash from the bloodstream the immunological soldiers that will win the day for us. Thus IgE, with its ability to release histamine-like chemicals, is not useless—far from it. This form of *controlled* immediate hypersensitivity is an essential element of the human defense.

The chemicals released from mast cells are meant to act *locally* and certainly not meant to have effects far removed from the site of the initiating events. But, as with so many things in life, there can be too much of a good thing. Too much IgE means that too many mast cells will explode; too much histamine will be released and the local effect will be exaggerated. The chemicals from the mast cells will find their way to other parts of the body.

As a group, the chemicals in mast cells tend to open blood vessels by causing the muscles surrounding them to relax, but the same chemicals have the *opposite* effects on muscles surrounding the airways, that is, the pipes that transport the air we inhale down into the lungs wherein oxygen is delivered to the blood.

The muscles of the airways go into spasm and breathing becomes difficult during a generalised allergic reaction, while at the same time the blood vessels may dilate excessively. Affected blood vessels in the skin will allow too much fluid to escape into the tissues, which consequently become stretched and then irritated by the chemicals therein. This accumulation of irritating fluid causes a swelling known popularly as a 'hive'; that is, an itchy red swelling which is technically known as urticaria.

So you can see that Von Pirquet, in the light of current knowledge, would have to modify his concept of useless allergy. It is only useless and harmful if overdone; properly controlled, it is a great system.

Even the uselessness of excessive IgE reactions is being challenged. Scientists have long pondered the unusual fact that up to twenty-four per cent of the world's population suffer from allergic reactions of one sort or another. Nature does not usually make such chronic and large mistakes. Over the eons, populations with inferior biological responses tend to disappear. Could immediate hypersensitivity therefore be an example of a biological tradeoff? Could Nature have found that potent IgE-mediated reactions protect us from something far worse than the discomfort of hay fever, asthma and hives?

There are a series of biological precedents for this form of accommodation. Here is one example. In certain parts of the world where malaria is a big problem, an enzyme deficiency is common. This deficiency produces a mild form of anemia that inconveniences the populace but that also protects its victims from getting malaria, a far worse problem than the anemia.

More than twenty studies in the literature claim that individuals who suffer from allergies experience less cancer than do others. This certainly would be a nice example of a biological tradeoff if it were true; unfortunately, many other studies in the literature deny the association. Nevertheless, some advantage to being 'atopic', the medical term used to describe the tendency to have too much IgE, may yet be revealed.

By carefully taking a history, a doctor may determine that hay fever symptoms are restricted to that six weeks of the year when ragweed pollen is predominant in the air. The patient may report that his itchy eyes, wheezing, stuffed-up nose etc., are really bothersome only during the summer or when he is at work. He is not allergic to summer work, but may well be allergic to the fungus that grows on the filters of the office air conditioner. Such organisms may be blown around the room with that nice refreshing cool air that you crave.

Someone may only have to get into the car of a cat fancier to have an attack of wheezing. Even if the cats are not in the car, as long as they have been there, they have left behind some dander, those tiny and therefore easily air-dispersed flakes of cat skin that cause so much trouble for the person allergic to this material.

Historical detective work is all important in getting to the basis of an allergy problem. Year-round allergies mean year-round exposure to the one or more things you react to. One of the most common causes of this problem is house dust or, more specifically, something contained in house dust.

Someone who is proud of the cleanliness of his or her home may notice that if the bed is made when the sun is shining through the window at the correct angle, millions of little particles are dispersed into the air. The same thing occurs every time anyone crossed a carpet or plonks into a well upholstered couch. House dust frequently contains fecal particles from an uninvited but common visitor to the home; the house dust mite.

In the average North American mattress, one can expect to find hundred of little ticklike creatures called mites. Several studies suggest that even more of the animals may be found in the mattresses of Europe. These little mites thrive on the privacy to be found inside your mattress and the warmth (sometimes heat) of the body or bodies lying on top.

The mites themselves do little harm, but relatively speaking they do produce many fecal particles. These would be harmless if it were not for the peculiarly fastidious nature of the mite. Unlike most other species, the mite wraps its feces in a gluey liquid material: that is, it bundles it up for disposal, so to speak. For those with the right (or wrong) genes, the coating around the feces is highly immunogenic. Problems develop when we breathe the coated particles into our airways where they can trigger off reactions mediated by IgE.

To make absolutely certain that you know how, for example, ragweed plant pollen could cause a blocked nose or indeed make a nose run like a tap, let us meet a sufferer. John, at thirty-six years of age, has suffered from seasonal rhinitis (inflammation inside the nose) for many years. For six weeks a year his nose is pretty well blocked.

We use our nose to discern flavor. The taste buds of our tongues are in reality useless to us in the subtle business of distinguishing a gourmet sauce from the everyday variety. Our tongue can distinguish the difference between sweetness, sourness and bitterness, etc., but it cannot subdifferentiate flavors. With your nose completely blocked, an apple or an onion tastes the same. Wonderful nerves in our nose *recognise* distinctive odors on which we depend for pleasure when eating and for alarm signalling in other situations, in a very immunological way. Individual nerve fibres ending in the nose have little projections extruding into the cavity of the nostril. Just as lymphocytes can recognise only one antigen, so also any one nerve cell can only recognise one odor. When a particular nerve recognises its 'odor', it sends an electric message to the brain and we 'taste' or 'smell' the odor that will consequently be conjured up in our brains. This wonderful distinguishing capacity is denied when the nose is blocked.

The nose is also used to add water to the air we inhale. Nature meant us to breathe through the nose. The rich blood supply to the nose, (which may make it bleed easily) and the mucous glands of the nose that contain so much moisture, mean that we can rapidly warm and humidify the air we inhale. The hairs inside the nose trap a great deal of airborne debris that should not enter the lungs. All in all, the nose is a most complicated, sophisticated and essential organ: hence, its removal from action is considerably more than a nuisance.

When ragweed pollen enters John's nose, some of it is absorbed through the vascular membrane of that organ. This can happen to all of us. The antigen is soon recognised by B cells but unfortunately for John they are programmed to make an excessive amount of IgE to this antigen. Subsequent inhalation of ragweed pollen into John's nose will set up a situation where the pollen, on being absorbed through the membrane of the nose, meets a great deal of already-formed IgE antibody. The IgE that is present on second and later exposures to ragweed is sitting on top of mast cells, as we have already described. Chemicals from mast cells are released once the ragweed interacts with the IgE. These chemicals will cause the copious blood vessels of the nose to swell or dilate. As they swell, the pores in the membrane will open up and much fluid will escape from the blood vessels into the surrounding tissues. This will force the delicate membranes of the nose to swell and an occlusion of the nostrils will follow. It is possible for the mucosa of the nose to swell so much that, having become heavy with water, the membranes will actually prolapse, forming what we call a nasal polyp. Such is the nature of allergic rhinitis.

John has trouble with ragweed because he makes too much IgE to an antigen of this particular pollen. His wife does not. She may well have some IgE against ragweed in her bloodstream and indeed even in her nose, but not enough to produce the excessive reaction that causes symptoms.

In determining which symptoms described by a patient are caused by an immediate hypersensitivity reaction, a physician must rely on his knowledge of the type of disturbances the various chemicals involved may cause and his detective skills. He can be helped considerably by using Von Pirquet's skin testing trick providing he knows the pitfalls. Many doctors who practise 'allergy', I must warn you, do not.

If you scratch into the skin a trace amount of something you suspect a patient may be allergic to, an immediate reaction will confirm your suspicions while a negative one throws doubt on the matter. We like to use scratch tests as opposed to injections into the skin) for two reasons. The injection of even small amounts of antigen into the skin of a subject who is extremely sensitised can provoke such a violent reaction that death may actually occur. Secondly, we are looking for extremes of sensitivity when we skin test a patient. As explained earlier a reaction is, in itself, not an abnormality. It is the extremes of the reaction that we seek. Normal people will not produce an immediately visible reaction to trace amounts of the material being investigated.

I can well remember as a young intern itching to do a little surgery on my own. On rare occasions the intern, who is of course, the lowest member of the medical team, will be allowed to suture a wound or perform some very minor surgical procedure. At the end of one very long operating day a surgeon turned to me and told me my big moment had arrived. The last patient on the list had a small wart-like polyp on his back which I could remove all on my own. All I had to do was to inject a little anesthetic around the area, cut out the lump and then put one or two stitches in place to stop the bleeding. Not exactly a heart transplant but I took it.

With only a pair of admiring nurses left to watch my skill I began to inject the local anesthetic into the back of the patient. I could not have injected more than a drop of fluid before the patient collapsed on the table and rapidly started to wheeze horribly and turn a deathly shade of pale. The patient had had an immediate hypersensitivity reaction to the local anesthetic. It took two days in the intensive care unit with all sorts of sophisticated machinery and drugs to get this patient back to normal. I had a very healthy respect for immediate hypersensitivity from that point on.

Very sensitive blood tests may now measure IgE antibodies to a whole array of antigens (or allergens, as they are often called in this context). The assays use radioactive isotopes which can be chemically attached to IgE antibodies and are very sensitive indeed, though not very easy to interpret.

I recently saw a wasted and pale IBM executive who had been referred to me for his terrible problem with allergies. The poor man had developed chronic hives six months earlier and since then had been almost unremittingly miserable because of the itching and swelling that constantly worried his eyes, hands and feet. His local doctor had referred him to an allergist who had ordered a myriad of IgE blood tests looking for antibodies to more than seventy different food substances as well as drugs, grasses, pollens, etc. Three thousand two hundred dollars later, the IBM executive was told the bad news. He had IgE antibodies to almost every food line for which tests had been done.

He immediately protested that he had never been allergic to anything in his life before and certainly could not relate his hives to eating. The allergist, however, assured him that all was now changed. An exclusion diet was devised for the poor man which allowed him to eat only rice, lettuce and some lamb. Everything he liked was banned.

Valiantly he struggled on, attempting to observe the diet for many months. During this time he lost weight, which he did not need to do, as well as his urticaria (hives). The doctor was gratified, the patient was not, because he felt that the cure was worse than the disease. A rebellious spirit arose within him and he sought a second opinion.

In talking to this man I learned that the doctor whom he had first consulted had relied on the blood tests exclusively rather than the story of the reactions which, as it turns out, contained important clues. I also learned that no attempt had been made to eliminate one food group at a time. After I questioned him closely, I was not convinced he needed to be on such a strict diet.

At the time his urticaria had developed he had been under great strain at work and I suspected that his problem might not be allergic at all. Not all urticaria, that is the abnormal dilation of blood vessels in the skin, is caused by IgE-related mechanisms. Slowly we returned this man to a normal diet and his urticaria did not return.

The moral in all this is that drastic treatment based on the exclusive use of these very sensitive blood tests is a mistake. The tests that pick up IgE antibody to various things are valuable in confirming suspicions based on history and skin testing and they supply us with a valuable research tool, but they are not ready for use in general practice.

In searching for an allergist, look for a doctor who is a diplomat of the allergy/immunology board, a sub-specialty group sanctioned by the American Medical Association to examine and then proclaim an individual's successful completion of training in this area. In other countries, check with the local college of physicians for ways of identifying individuals who have successfully completed training in immunology.

I believe it is particularly important to avoid those doctors who practise ear, nose and throat surgery but who throw in 'allergy' as an extra. Unfortunately, there is an ever-increasing number of such individuals in North America & elsewhere. Although there are some exceptions, most doctors who are basically ENT surgeons are very inadequate when it comes to handling allergic diseases. Time and time again I have had patients referred to me who have been completely mismanaged by these individuals.

For many ENT surgeons, allergy is a lucrative sideline. Be particularly wary of the doctor who tells you how lucky you are that he actually has in his office a machine that will do the blood tests we described above. These tests, which are unlikely to be interpreted correctly by the untrained observer, may cost you a fortune.

One of the major problems in the allergy business is only slowly being solved. Relatively few substances that cause allergic reactions have actually been purified.

Imagine you have an allergic reaction every time you eat tomatoes. In loose unscientific terminology, you might say you are allergic to 'tomatoes'. What you actually mean, of course, is that you respond to something in the complex makeup of a tomato. This may not even be present in the undigested tomato; it may turn up in your body only after your metabolism has got to work in breaking down the chemicals present when you first swallowed the tomato. For this reason, allergy tests that use crude extracts of a particular food tend to be very unreliable.

Recently a team of excellent immunologists from San Antonio, Texas, examined scientifically all the available tests to diagnose food allergy, including those already described. They concluded that the only way to diagnose food allergy was by careful history taking, followed by the removal from the diet of food or groups of food about which one had become suspicious. If the patient improved, this could be followed by a challenge, with a suspicious item or items being reintroduced into the diet. Done carefully under controlled conditions, this is a safe procedure that may prevent someone from being unnecessarily deprived of some of life's great pleasures. What all this boils down to is that patients with suspected food allergies need careful assessment and management by experienced physicians who understand the mechanisms involved and the limitations of our present knowledge.

It is possible and indeed likely that in rare cases a patient may develop severe symptoms after eating something specific via a mechanism that has nothing to do with allergy. Food is nothing more than a currently acceptable bunching of chemicals with nutritional or appetite-satisfying properties. Some individuals' metabolism (body chemistry) may be different from that of most people and their reaction to the ingestion of, say, apple juice may be very different from yours and mine.

Sometimes the ingestion of a particular substance by such people may lead to the release of some of the chemicals that IgE can also release. In this case, however, the release is not activated through an immunological mechanism.

A few years ago I was involved as an 'expert witness' in a tragic case which was the subject of litigation. A medical mistake resulted in the death of a mother and a medical career.

Susan was a thirty-three-year-old mother of three. She was generally well but was being investigated for abnormally painful periods associated with severe headaches. Before the fulltime demands of motherhood, Susan had been a nurse and she suspected that a growth in her uterus had something to do with the problem. While under investigation, her period began and by 11 a.m. on the morning of its second day she was so uncomfortable that she took herself and her three young children to the emergency room at her local hospital. Here she was seen immediately by the nurse who filled out a brief medical history chart.

To the routine question, 'Are you allergic to anything?' Susan replied, 'Yes, I am allergic to aspirin.' At fifteen, she had been given aspirin for an attack of flulike symptoms and developed a rash and wheezing. A doctor had told her she must not take aspirin again. She was eventually seen by the doctor who listened to her story, examined her and came to his conclusion: this patient, he reasoned, was being investigated by a competent gynecologist; his job was to relieve her present discomfort, nothing more.

As is not uncommon in busy emergency rooms, he had four to five other patients in various cubicles simultaneously and he flitted from one to the other in attempts to be efficient. The nurses' notes for each patient were on his desk, paperwork to be completed in a quiet moment.

The young doctor in question was training to be a specialist in internal medicine and was supporting himself and a young wife and child by helping out in the emergency room. He was knowledgeable, but inexperienced. He prescribed a relaxant-analgesic preparation for Susan and at 2.16 p.m. his patient was discharged from the emergency room at the hospital. The preparation he prescribed contained, among other things, significant amounts of aspirin. At 2.35 p.m. Susan had her prescription filled by a pharmacist. By 3.15 she had taken the first tablet and, after leaving the children with her next door neighbor, had sunk gratefully onto her bed to await relief.

At approximately 4.30 p.m., the young doctor at the hospital was catching up with his paperwork. As he filled in Susan's forms he recalled the case and noticed underlined, the nurse's warning: 'Patient allergic to aspirin'. After his initial shock at realising his mistake and the possible consequences of what he had done, he reassured himself that no real harm would probably come to the patient. He clearly must call, however, and tell her not to take any more of the tablets.

No one answered the telephone at Susan's house. Even though he thought it most likely that the unanswered telephone meant that she was out, some uneasy premonition made him call at her address after he finished his roster at 5.30 p.m. Susan was dead and had been so since approximately 4 p.m. A post-mortem examination revealed that the cause of her death was consistent with acute bronchospasm; following the ingestion of the aspirin, she had suffocated. Reasonably under the circumstances, Susan's husband sued the hospital and the doctor and a considerable amount of money was awarded to the family, but it could have been of little consolation.

I told you the story about the aspirin because there is no evidence that in that particular type of reaction IgE antibody is involved at all. When Susan said she was allergic to aspirin, she was not being scientifically accurate. After ingestion into our bodies, a number of chemicals alter various biological pathways on which we rely. In some patients, as we discussed earlier, these alterations lead to the release of those very same chemicals that affect our blood vessels and airways in an allergic reaction; however, they cause the damage directly, rather than relying on anti-body.

Aspirin affects some pathways in the brain, enabling us to relieve pain, but it is also very useful as an anti-inflammatory agent. Whenever you have painful red and hot swellings in your body, for example, in the case of arthritis, aspirin is often useful. This drug is able to produce these anti-inflammatory effects by blocking the metabolic pathways that lead to the development of those chemicals that actually produce the inflammation.

The trouble with a number of drugs is that they do not know when to stop. In other words, unblocking one metabolic pathway that, for example, may make your joints feel better if you have arthritis may also simultaneously block a second pathway or perhaps even stimulate a second pathway that produces harmful effects. The significance of these potentially harmful effects may be clinically important in only a few individuals. This is what can happen when aspirin is ingested. A small number of people are so sensitive to the drug that while it produces the normal aspirin effects in them, it also leads to the accumulation in the body of chemicals involved in allergic-type reactions. These chemicals can make blood vessels dilate and airways constrict. Immunology does not come into the story at all.

The same mechanism can occur with a number of food preservatives and dyes. For example, the food preservative tartrazine and the red and yellow dyes we find in so many of our foods today can cause these problems for an individual who is particularly sensitive to these compounds.

Because of their knowledge of such situations, physicians and scientists must keep an open mind on the possibility that some bizarre symptomatology which we occasionally have described to us by our patients is in fact biochemically induced by that individual's particular metabolic sensitivity to some ingested substance. It is vitally important, however, that the physician be extremely objective about such a situation. While it is necessary to acknowledge that such problems exist, albeit rarely, one must be extremely careful not to explain away genuine psychological problems by postulating such mechanisms.

This problem is becoming increasing serious in a number of Western countries, particularly North America. A number of misguided or unscrupulous individuals are making a considerable amount of money from seriously psychiatrically disturbed patients by telling them that their problems are related to allergic reactions to things in the environment. In other words, they are supplying an organic reason for the bizarre symptomatology of a number of patients who would much rather believe this than face the fact that they are mentally disturbed. Of course, some people have very unusual biochemical pathways within their bodies that may make them extremely sensitive to environmental factors but that cause most of us no problem at all.

The following case illustrate the extremes to which unscientific thinking can go, and the financial and medical hazards than can follow.

Rebecca is twenty-nine years old and lives in New York City. Intelligent, attractive and well educated, she has not worked for a number of years, ostensibly because she cannot find a job. She is a trained social worker who has researched the problems of paroled prisoners and their integration back into society. Rebecca's childhood was not happy, though, unfortunately, not really extraordinary. She had an inadequate mother, a drunken bully of a father and a brother on drugs; all these things caused her much distress. Since the age of fifteen, she has suffered from seasonal allergic rhinitis and depression.

In 1980, Rebecca developed a most unusual medical problem: an allergy to Avery Fisher Hall in New York City. As a music lover, this was a real problem for her; many of the city's major concerts are held in this hall.

To be accurate, Rebecca's problem was in the foyer of Avery Fisher Hall: she could not make it into the hall proper. Within seconds of walking through the door of the foyer, she became weak, dizzy and breathless and sank to the floor unconscious. When she visited two or three apartments belonging to friends, the same thing happened. In discussing this matter with her undoubtedly very concerned friends, she was eventually advised to seek the advice of a 'clinical ecologist' practicing in New York City. This she did and was told she must enter a clinic for prolonged testing. She went to a southern state for two weeks of investigation at a clinic designed specifically to study such problems.

I met Rebecca a few months later in my outpatients' clinic at Yale University. When I entered the examination room with my nurse and greeted the patient routinely, there was no answer, and indeed no movement of any sort from Rebecca. The nurse and I approached her and spoke to her again and, with an obvious effort, she slowly moved her hand, extended her finger and pointed to the pocket of her jacket. The nurse removed from her pocket a note and a small bottle containing a clear fluid and dropper. The note was brief but informative: in case of catatonia, place three drops of histamine under the tongue.

Catatonia involves rigid immobilisation of muscles. Rebecca slowly opened her mouth and it was obvious what she expected us to do. We dutifully placed three drops of the fluid from the bottle marked histamine under her tongue and a miracle occurred. Within two seconds she relaxed, smiled and said hello.

After that most unusual start to her interview, a full history was taken. Rebecca had come to see me because she was still not well after her trip to the southern clinic but at least she now knew that her problem was due to T cell dysfunction; could I help?

It turned out that she had been admitted twice to the clinical ecology unit in the southern state. On the first visit they told her after $4800 worth of tests that she had total allergy syndrome. Rebecca was allergic to everything.

She had been discharged with thirty-two bottles, from which she was to inject tiny amounts of matter into herself.

Rebecca came home, got worse not better, developing these strange attacks of stiffness, and returned to the clinic for further help. After one week, one of the clinic specialists told her that she had the most severe form of this problem. They explained that her really severe case of total allergy syndrome was caused by a lack of normal T cells. She discharged herself, apparently with great difficulty, returned to New York and saw me.

On that first visit, she emptied the contents of her brown bag onto my desk. The thirty-two bottles of injectable extracts appeared, all hand labelled and made at the clinic. There were also vitamins and amino acid preparations, including one made from the testicles of a New Zealand bull.

Rebecca was clearly a psychiatrically disturbed young woman and I am pleased to tell you that with help from a psychiatrist at a major university in New York City, she is employed and almost symptom-free at this writing.

We have talked about how important history-taking is in any encounter with a medical problem, particularly in the search for potential allergens. It did not take long to find out that Rebecca's fiance had disengaged himself one night right there in the foyer of the Avery Fisher Hall. You don't have to be Freud to work out the rest of the story.

At this point, I think we should say a few words about the disease asthma. There is much confusion on this important subject; between 4 and 8 per cent of the population are made miserable because of this problem at some time.

The word asthma is derived from two Greek words meaning 'difficult breathing' and if you have ever seen a patient suffering from an attack of asthma, you will surely agree that this is a very conservative name for this horrible condition. Asthma is one of the major health problems in the world today, causing a great deal of suffering to many people, both children and adults, and costing billions of dollars in lost productivity. Particularly disturbing is the fact that in many countries, the death rate from asthma, after decreasing for a number of years, is rising again.

We have already mentioned the fact that blood vessels are surrounded by a circular coat of muscle that can contract and therefore narrow in diameter or relax and increase in diameter. The same is true of the bronchial tree. Air breathed in through the nose or mouth must travel to the lungs by means of a network of pipes that together make up the bronchial tree. The first part of this branching system is called the trachea, and you can feel this by putting your hand on your neck just above the little notch you have at the bottom of your throat. Here you can feel the hard rings of cartilage which make the trachea the big patent pipe that it is. As the bronchial tree branches and takes the air downwards into the lungs, the cartilage that supports the major airways disappears and the diameter of the lumen is controlled by muscles arranged in exactly the same way as they are around blood vessels.

When an individual suffers from episodic attacks wherein there is spasming (narrowing) of the small airways, the condition known as asthma (reversible airways obstruction) occurs.

While the mechanics and physiology of breathing are very complicated, we can easily present the basic facts. When taking a breath we inhale into our lungs air containing about 20 per cent oxygen. The lungs extract the oxygen and deliver it to the red blood cells. They whisk the oxygen around the body, delivering it to muscles and tissues that could not survive more than a few minutes without this precious commodity. It is obviously necessary to breathe out before we can breathe in again, but Nature does not waste the expiratory part of the breathing cycle. When we breathe out we expel the gas carbon dioxide from our lungs and our bodies. Carbon dioxide is a by-product of many metabolic processes in the body and it must be regularly cleared from our system. If it is not, it forms an acid in the bloodstream which is extremely dangerous.

When you take a deep breath you expand your chest, and the pressure inside your lungs decreases so that there is a natural tendency for your airways to open up. This is a fine arrangement because that is exactly the time when you want the maximum amount of air to go down into your lungs. As you breathe out, the reverse happens; the pressure in your airways increases and it is normal for the bronchial tree to narrow during expiration.

Patients who suffer from asthma have airways that are too narrow so that not only do they have trouble in getting enough air into their lungs, they may find it impossible to get the carbon dioxide out. As they try to exhale, their airways narrow but to such a point that frequently no air movement is possible and air that is devoid of oxygen and therefore useless is trapped in their lungs. The brain, sensing that it is not getting enough oxygen to enrich the circulating blood, sends all sorts of panic signals to the lungs and chest. Patients begin to fight for more air and in their struggles often become exhausted.

The important question, of course, is why do some people have airways that spasm? Why do the muscles surrounding the bronchial tree of asthma victims try and suffocate them? In order to understand the answers to these questions, one must appreciate the fact that Nature loves to control most things in the body using a tug-of-war system. Right now, your heart is beating at a certain rate which represents the net result of two sets of simultaneously active but opposing nervous stimuli. One set of nerves is trying to speed up your heart while the other is trying to slow it down; the balance between these two opposing tug-of-war teams determines your heart rate.

Exactly the same is true of the muscles controlling the diameter of your airways. In any given moment, signals are passing down nerves to release chemicals that instruct the muscle cells of the airways to relax. Simultaneously, however, messages are coming from other nerves that tell the very same cells to contract. The tone of the muscle, which is the net influence of the two opposing forces, determines just how open or closed your airways will be at any given moment.

Asthma is caused by a defect in the control of the muscle cells of the airways. These muscles possess little receptors on their membranes which can interact with or interpret the chemical messages released by the nerves that want the muscle to relax. These are known as Beta receptors. Quite distinct receptors accept messages telling the muscle cells to contract. When a tug-of-war team is evenly balanced, one side will win handsomely when an extra man is placed on that side. Exactly the same result will occur if one man is dropped from the opposition. In either case the result will be a movement in the same direction. With this analogy in mind, you can imagine that asthma might be due to increased sensitivity to the signals that cause the muscles to constrict, or equally to a loss of sensitivities to the chemicals that tell the muscles to relax. In most cases, the latter situation seems to be responsible for the asthmatic's problems. The muscle cells are not particularly responsive to signals trying to activate the Beta receptors. Whether such receptors are damaged in patients with asthma or simply present but in insufficient numbers to do the job properly is currently a matter for some debate. The result, however, is quite clear. Even normal stimulation from those chemicals that cause muscles to constrict will not be opposed by the normal counterbalancing forces that stop constriction. The net result will be airways which are significantly narrowed.

It is important to have these mechanisms discussed because asthma is widely held to be an allergic disease, i.e., it is caused by mechanisms involving IgE antibody. The truth is that asthma is a disorder of the airways and allergic reactions around those airways, because they release chemicals which cause muscles in the airways to constrict, can trigger off an attack of asthma. The basic defect must be present before an allergic reaction can produce bronchospasm.

A patient with asthma is like a man walking along the edge of a dangerously high cliff. While he is walking along the edge of that cliff and has not tumbled over, he is perfectly safe. The closer he is to the edge of the cliff, however, the closer he is to danger. If he is teetering on the edge of the cliff, one good push and tragedy could develop. In other words even when a patient with asthma appears to be perfectly well his airways will be narrower than yours or mine. He no longer has any reserve capacity as he cannot function normally with any further narrowing of this airways. Under such circumstances, an allergic reaction will precipitate an asthma attack, push him over the cliff.

With the vulnerability caused by these imbalances in the airways, an asthmatic patient may have an attack precipitated by emotion, pollution in the air, exercise, sudden exposure to cold air, infection, certain drugs and allergic reactions. Modern therapy is designed to identify triggering factors that can bring on an attack of asthma and if possible remove them from the patient's environment. This is combined with treatment of the underlying condition. In this day and age this, basically, involves attempts to make the Beta receptor more sensitive to the chemicals that normally activate it, while administering drugs to the airways that stimulate the receptor. The disease is such a significant problem that I feel I must add a few notes for those of you who are victims of asthma to help you determine whether or not you are getting the best therapy currently available.

You are in good hands if your doctor has been at pains to explain the mechanisms that I have just described so that you can feel comfortable that you understand what the disease is all about; if he emphasises that modern treatment concentrates on delivering the necessary drugs via the airways rather than through injected or swallowed medication; if, in putting you on inhaled medication, he has thoroughly checked more than once to make sure the technique you are using to inhale the medicine is correct; if he gives you a small peak expiratory flow meter that you keep at home and use so you can determine for yourself what progress you are making with your disease. These little gadgets measure how narrow or wide are your airways, and tell you such things as whether or not you are responding to the medicine you have been asked to inhale. A fall in the reading on the meter suggests you are heading for a severe attack of asthma, an observation that allows you to alert your doctor. Your doctor should also have ensured that blood levels have been taken frequently to determine the right dose of theophylline which you need to give you maximum therapeutic response (theophylline is a drug which has the ability to dilate the bronchial tree) and, realising that your problem may be brought on by exercise or cold air, he should have explained to you that you can prevent these attacks by using an inhaled stimulant of the Beta receptor before beginning exercise or venturing into the cold air. He should have told you that only in the most unusual circumstances are desensitisation attempts (shots) warranted for the patient with asthma.

The mention of desensitisation needs further explanation. Desensitisation is a technique that has been used for many years by allergists in an attempt to reduce IgE-mediated sensitivity. The technique, which is practiced on millions of people every week of every year, involves repeated injections of tiny doses of the allergen thought to be causing a patient's symptoms, over a long period of time.

Why should this technique be considered useful? Until recently the most popular theory as to how desentisisation might work involved the production after the 'shots' of IgG antibody to the allergen in question. When natural exposure to the allergen occurred there would be, sitting there waiting for it, another antibody in the body which could compete for the allergen with the IgE sitting on top of mast cells. If there is enough IgE in your circulation to pounce on the allergen as soon as it enters your body, it may be able to bind it all up, so that little was around to trigger the IgE on the mast cells in the tissues.

This was quite a logical theory and, in fact, there may be some truth in the suggestion, but it is certainly not the complete answer. Very recent studies strongly suggest that on occasions immunoregulatory T cells that can control IgE production to a specific allergen may be stimulated by the desensitising injections. This may allow the patient to regain control of his IgE production. Remember, we stated at the beginning of this discussion on allergy that the thermostat determining how much IgE you will or will not produce lives within the genetic apparatus of the T cells.

Unfortunately it is very difficult to ensure that desensitisation of any patient will result in success. The technique may produce serious results as we are dealing with a very powerful system. If too much allergen is given, an allergic reaction of dangerous proportions can be triggered right in the doctor's office. Nevertheless, in skilled hands, the risks associated with it are quite acceptable and the cost-benefit ratio needs to be closely examined until we can more scientifically formulate the right dose for an individual. This will become much easier as more purified allergens become available. You will find that most clinical immunologists working in a university centre are very conservative in their approach to desensitisation and tend to put an enormous amount of emphasis on finding the allergen that is causing the trouble and then helping their patient to avoid it. If this is not possible then reliance is placed on the use of pharmacological approaches that will block the consequences of IgE mediated reactions.

At this writing I can say confidently that we are good at desensitising people to things like ragweed and now cat dander, and that beneficial effects can be expected when the allergens causing the problems for a specific patient are clearly identifiable and few in number. If your skin lights up like Times Square on New Year's Eve when you are skin tested, it is extremely unlikely that desensitisation will be able to control your problems. You have simply developed allergies to too many different things.

There certainly are indications for attempting to desensitise people with allergic problems and a classic situation involves sensitivity to bee and wasp venom. A number of deaths occur each year from massive allergic reaction following a bee sting. People can become extremely sensitive to the venom of these insects. But the interesting fact is that more people die of their fear of being stung than the reality of being stung. Statistics show that people who know they are allergic to bee and wasp venom frequently become terrified when they find themselves in a moving car accompanied by a bee or wasp, and they are likely to have an accident.

Initial attempts at desensitising people to bee and wasp venom relied on a crude extract from the insects. The bodies of a particular type of bee or wasp suspected of causing the problem were literally crushed and the fluid squeezed from the hapless creatures was diluted appropriately and injected into the patient. Results were not very encouraging. However, far purer venom extracts are now available from various bees and wasps and it is possible to skin test patients to find out which particular variety of insect is a problem for them. Results of desensitisation using venom are very encouraging.

In general, desensitisation has a much better track record in controlling symptoms referrable to the nose and eyes rather than the chest. You are more likely to benefit from desensitisation therapy if allergic rhinitis is your problem, rather than asthma.

Diagnosing genuine allergic reactions to food is also a very difficult business. If at the first bite of food cooked in peanut oil your tongue and pharynx swell, there is not much doubt about the diagnosis. But it is not easy when the reactions to food are delayed, as they frequently are, and the further the time of reaction from the time of ingestion the more difficult is the historical reconstruction of the possible precipitating events.

Many 'allergists' claim to be able to diagnose your food allergy with pinpoint precision. As with our IBM executive discussed already, they may tell you that you are allergic to many things which, in reality, cause you no trouble at all. The tests they use represent some of the worst examples of empiricism in modern medical practice. They vary from 'cytotoxic testing' wherein some of your blood cells are taken and exposed to food extracts, only to die if you are allergic to the food, through to challenges where you eat a food and have your nose swabbed at hourly intervals. The appearance of certain cells in the nose, some would suggest, indicates that you are allergic to that food. All such tests are useless and you should avoid any doctor or paramedical personnel who has any faith in this approach.

If your allergist has explained all these facts to you, you are probably in good hands. If he has asked you to vacuum up some of the dust on your floor so that you may bring it to his office and have him prepare an extract to use for desensitisation purposes, you are in trouble. If he makes such an extract and asks you to put it under your tongue, you are dealing with a physician who has drifted far away from the mainstream of modern immunological thought. If he has told you that all those colds you get, especially those sore throats you had last winter, may be due to allergies to bacterial products and he is therefore desensitising you with 'bacterial vaccines', run a mile to your nearest board of certified allergists and get some informed help. All these approaches are distressingly common in many countries of the world.

One further aspect of allergic disease must be discussed which concerns that wonderful immunomodulator known as breast milk. Nature is faced with a dilemma in protecting the intestinal tract and the upper airways of the newborn baby from bacterial infection. The baby's immune system must mature over the first few months of life, learning first how to make IgM then IgG before it can make IgA, that antibody which protects our delicate mucous membranes. In order to make sure that IgA is available to the intestinal tract of the baby, mothers are meant to breast feed their infants. Nature has made specific arrangements to ensure that adequate amounts of IgA antibodies that can protect the baby's intestinal tract are in breast milk.

In recent years it has become clear that there is an association between a natural inability to produce IgA and allergies to a number of things, particularly to certain foods. Recent research has revealed that much of the sensitisation to such things as gluten, soy and milk proteins which have caused so many people so much trouble, occur during the first year of life. Apart from the ability of IgA to protect us from viral and bacterial infections, these molecules may also have an important role to play in protecting us from developing allergies. Abundant quantities of IgA in the intestinal tract can certainly minimise the absorption across the mucous membranes of gluten, soy and milk proteins and probably many other things as well.

In the absence of IgA, these proteins, which we normally do not absorb in an allergenic form, stimulate IgE production and the allergic cascade commences.

Researchers in Scandinavia have shown that a baby who is born to parents both of whom have 'allergies' had a very high chance of developing severe allergic symptoms before the age of one. That risk, however, is very significantly reduced if the baby is breast fed for the first year of life. Apparently, keeping IgA available to the infant's intestinal tract during that first year blocks the absorption of material that can sensitise the child. As we mentioned earlier, a number of milk banks have been established in Scandinavia so that milk is available for 'therapeutic purposes'.

Let us conclude on a positive note. Those of you who find immediate hypersensitivity reactions to be producing symptoms that interfere with the quality of your lives should be heartened to know that competent clinical immunologists are available to help with most problems in this area. Certainly major advances in immunology and pharmacology over the next few years will greatly improve the management of that 'useless allergy' so clearly recognised by Von Pirquet at the beginning of this century.

8 | The painful subject of autoimmunity

T HE man in question had brutally attacked his wife after a domestic argument.

A psychiatrist was discussing this case with his fourth-year medical students who had been present when he had examined the man. The students, who had seen photos of the wife's condition immediately after the assault, were not sympathetic to the man's protestation of remorse and promises of change. They wanted him locked away for years, and trotted forth newspaper accounts they could recall where men such as this one, when dealt with leniently by the courts, went on to do worse damage to their victims, perhaps even killing some of them.

The psychiatrist tried to bring a more professional, dispassionate perspective to the case. The man was clearly not psychotic; he could distinguish reality from fantasy. Nowhere in his testing did he reveal disturbances of thought patterns that would suggest that his personality was hovering on that dangerous tightrope that separates the merely neurotic from the frankly psychotic. Although the man was not particularly intelligent he knew right from wrong and had himself and his aggressive tendencies under control at most times.

All his episodes of violence had followed the consumption of a significant amount of alcohol at a time of family financial crisis.

'There are thousands of men and women like that one out in the real world,' the psychiatrist pointed out to the students. 'They don't have strong personalities but with help many such men can gain better control of themselves, especially if they are carefully watched by an emotionally indifferent, authoritarian and potentially punitive third party. Probation, supervised help for his drinking problems and family counselling might save this man. Oh sure, the failure rate is high, but what are the alternatives? Lock him away for many years in case he does not reform? As a society, we must generate universally acceptable constraints that reinforce the need for self-control.'

The above case and discussion are purely hypothetical, although one knows that they are only too likely to mimic real-life situations. But the analogies between the incidents related above and the deviations of an immune system that is attacking self will, I hope, become obvious. When we talk of autoimmunity, we are discussing a situation in which less than perfect genetic starting material combined with environmental stress, can lead to a breakdown in self-control that can produce disease.

Among the four to six hundred billion lymphocytes that secure your body are some that are potentially 'sociopathic', in this sense, I suppose you could say 'organopathic'. Just as with human personality, there are numerous genetic permutations and combinations that affect the performance of lymphocytes.

We know that each and every lymphocyte is capable of recognising only one antigen, using its membrane receptor for the task. This receptor has a three-dimensional spatial configuration that allows it to act as a lock into which only one key can fit properly. The potential problem with all this lymphocyte individualism is that Nature has generated cells that can recognise 'us' as well as foreignness. Just as many cells recognise your own kidney cells as can recognise a herpes virus.

At one stage in the evolution of immunological knowledge it was thought or rather presumed that, under normal circumstances, Nature would have instituted a system for eliminating cells with 'attack potential' for self. This 'clonal abortion' (killing of a family of autoreactive cells) would presumably occur as the cells were formed. As a result of this smart move, we would then have no chance of developing an autoimmune disease in which an organ could be viciously attacked and damaged by an 'organopathic' cell.

When it became obvious that such tissue attacks did occur, the theory was modified. It seemed that some of us were unfortunate enough to lack the ability to induce clonal abortion and so these potential 'time bombs' survived in our bodies.

None of us, it turns out, aborts those T cells that can recognise self tissues. We humans must accept the fact that millions of cells in our body would attack us mercilessly if they followed their basic inclinations. For our survival, therefore, they need to know that this is not the right thing for them to do, so they may exert a measure of self-control over their auto-aggressive natures. They need to be aware that big brother is watching them and urging passivity. It is the same situation that faces our wife basher; self control and third-party regulatory pressures offer the best chances of avoiding dangerous escapes from acceptable behavior.

Lymphocytes can only recognise, for example, a specific section of our nervous system because they have been given the receptor to do so by genetic selection. A wife basher has less of an excuse for attacking her than does our auto-aggressive lymphocyte for attacking the nervous system. Nevertheless, these cells are breaking carefully laid down rules if they do attack us. Let us examine the controls that the immunological society places upon them.

Our immune system has to deal with a compromise situation since the system is not yet perfected, just as human society has to deal with the far from Utopian makeup of human interactions. Major control of auto-aggression results from a simple fact that we have dealt with many times: in any immune reaction, a pivotal step involves permissive signals being given by one type of T cell; the inducer or helper T cell. If this cell says 'attack' then a veritable army of cells with different weaponry spring into action.

All day every day, T cells from this inducer family look at our own tissues, recognise them and decide not to attack. This crucial, and of course, correct decision means that those other T and B cells that can recognise our own tissues do not get the 'go ahead' signals they need to attack. All remains peaceful and our organs go about their business unassailed.

Why do T cells that recognise us, using a perfectly legitimate and specific membrane receptor, not attack 'self' while others, appearing to take part in exactly the same sort of interaction but with 'foreignness', launch into battle? There are, as you would probably imagine, numerous reasons for this restraint as it would be very dangerous to have all our self-control eggs in the one basket.

Generally speaking, our T cells 'tolerate' the presence of self. This tolerance can be divided into two types, passive and active. Passive tolerance is 'self-contained'. Imagine a stray dog has adopted your family. You do not really want a dog but the kids want to keep it. You debate the issue, shrug your shoulders, smile at the kids and the dog moves closer to the fire. That is passive tolerance. On the other hand you may dearly wish to reject the mangy dog and would do so if a superior authority did not intervene. 'Henry,' says mother firmly, 'the children will be broken-hearted if you do not let them keep that dog; don't you even think of getting rid of it.' That is active tolerance. The dog immediately curls up in your favorite chair.

In immunological terms, many T inducer cells that can recognise our own tissues are passively tolerant. During fetal life when immature, indeed simplistic cells are grouping themselves to form our early tissues and organs, T cells are genetically instructed to look at those developing structures. If they recognise them during the critical phase of fetal development they are instructed by genetic messages from within their nucleus to be tolerant. Before eighteen weeks of fetal life, cells are instructed that *anything they recognise* is 'self' and therefore it must be left alone. During fetal life the only thing around to look at should be 'us', and therefore this instruction should ensure that tolerance develops only to self. Since many of those T cells present at, say, ten weeks of fetal life will still be working sixty years later, the educational message given to the youngsters can control autoimmune tendencies for most of life.

Simultaneously and, some feel, more importantly, immunoregulatory T cells are active during fetal life that are taught to recognise self and then secrete specific chemicals that will actively prevent a T inducer cell from coming off the appropriate tracks should it ever be so inclined. This is very much *active* tolerance.

Tolerance can be infectious. Apparently new T cells that are derived from the thymus later in life receive signals from both the passively tolerant and actively tolerant cells.

We do not worry too much about the B cells in this system; they live only for a few days. It would be a waste of biological energy to teach them tolerance as their life is too short and they cannot do anything without T cell help anyway.

As you can imagine, just how well all of this works and its ability to function throughout life, depends on the quality of the genetic program setting it up in the first place. The quality of this information varies from individual to individual, as with everything human. Some people have superb control of the potentially lethal time bombs inside them, others have a tenuous hold on auto-aggression.

We are beginning to learn how to recognise these latter folk and that is an important development in preventative medicine. Weaker than normal genetic control of potential auto reactivity leaves us walking through life on a biological tightrope rather than down the middle of a broad pedestrian esplanade. People on tightropes can fall off spontaneously, but can also easily be pushed off their centre of balance. Much of human disease results from an interaction between 'second-class' genetic information and environmental circumstances.

Let me explain by giving an example. Diabetes is one of the most common and most serious diseases to afflict man. In its more severe forms, which tragically most frequently affect the young (sometimes even babies), the pancreas, the gland that secretes the hormone insulin, is the victim of auto-aggression.

The pancreas has two important functions. It produces chemicals that help us digest our food. These chemicals are squirted into our duodenum when we eat. We can live without them, but we cannot live without the literally vital production from specific beta cells within the gland; the hormone insulin.

Insulin is vital for many metabolic processes in our body, the most obvious of which is the pumping of sugar into our cells. Without insulin, the sugar dams up in our blood where it is useless and can have dangerous effects on the brain and other tissues. But much more is involved than that. Without insulin our bodies age prematurely; a forty-year-old diabetic looks like a sixty-five-year-old non-diabetic. When diabetes occurs in childhood, life expectancy can be reduced by as much as twenty-seven years. Children frequently develop premature hardening of the arteries, leading to heart attacks, blindness and severe kidney disease. Cataracts tend to form in the eyes and all the sugar in the blood and urine make the patient more susceptible to infection; bacteria love sugar. Even with the most careful attention by the patient and doctor to the injection of insulin and general health matters, the diabetic must face many problems.

Slowly over a period of months or more often years, patients with diabetes have their beta cells destroyed by their own T cells; a drastic example of autoimmunity. No pain is associated with the destruction and by the time the patient comes to the doctor with the first symptoms, 80 per cent of the beta cells have already been destroyed. Even while we are working hard to develop means of transplanting the pancreas we are very interested in an even more attractive solution to the problem. We are attempting to perfect ways of detecting individuals experiencing an autoimmune attack on the pancreas before serious permanent damage has been done. Having done this we must try and get those cells back on the straight and narrow path that is non-reactivity to self. Call off the attack on the pancreas, and diabetes will not develop.

Picking up potential diabetics in a phase where they are still well is possible because of our ability to seek genetic markers that make us suspicious that self-control may not be all we might desire.

You will recall that we humans all have biological trademarks that we display on the surface of our cells. They proudly proclaim 'me', that almost unique individual. These proteins are well displayed on white blood cells so we refer to the system as the HLA system, *h*uman *l*eucocyte (white blood cell) *a*ntigen system. In an earlier chapter, we discussed the fact that these cell markers are what make transplants so difficult.

The eight major and many more minor self antigens were not put there by the great immunologist in the sky to make transplantation difficult; they are there to help our immune system distinguish between self and foreignness. Remember, we will not attack anything until we look for those HLA antigens.

With the transplantation era came the development of the technology for tissue-typing people for their eight major HLA antigens. Using this information, perfect matches could be sought for transplantation purposes.

With many profiles being generated among both candidates for transplantation and potential donors, an astute Frenchman made an astounding observation; some of these HLA profiles seemed to turn up repeatedly in people with certain diseases. Sometimes only one of the eight major antigens seem to be associated with the disease (or sometimes unusual resistance to a disease); in other cases a constellation of HLA antigens seemed to be linked in some unknown way to a specific illness.

With the work that has gone on since those pioneering observations, we can report that we now know of more than one hundred diseases that seem to be associated in one way or another to an HLA profile. Such genetic profiles can supply you with better predictive information than you will ever get from reading your horoscope.

Now the big question raised by those observations was: Why should the presence, sometimes on every cell in your body (remember we use leucocytes for testing only for convenience) have anything to do with your getting a disease in one organ, such as psoriasis which affects the skin, arthritis which affects the joints, cancer, diabetes, etc.?

Well, the diseases have nothing to do with the HLA antigens themselves (although for a while people thought certain ones might act as receptors for viruses, etc.). No, it is a matter of association.

If you are in a long dark alley of 11th Avenue in New York and into the opposite end of the alley comes one kid who looks like a member of a tough neighborhood gang, you would not be surprised to find four seconds later that ten or twelve more members of the gang come swinging into the lane. The first kid may be harmless but he tends to keep company with a gang that is anything but harmless. You do not need to see the whole gang to know trouble could be on the way; just a glimpse of the first kid and you move right on. He keeps bad company.

Some HLA genes tend to mix in immunologically disreputable company. These HLA genes, which produce the antigens we detect by our tissue-typing, are harmless, but their presence indicates that on the sixth chromosome lurks a group of bad immunoregulatory genes that tend to allow disease processes such as autoimmunity to occur.

Now, of course, the kid from the gang could be followed into the alley on some occasions by the Salvation Army band. He is not the villain. Seeing a certain HLA antigen does not mean a definite propensity for a certain disease, it just increases the likelihood.

This association is much stronger, however, with certain profiles. One such profile consists of cells displaying D locus genes known as 3 and 4. This is a bad combination, increasing the risk that disease-causing genes for many problems are present, including multiple sclerosis, rheumatoid arthritis and diabetes. About 30 per cent of people in the world are unaffected by the presence of DR3 and DR4, however.

The reason that certain HLA genes and genes coding regulatory performance stick together through many generations needs explaining. Chromosomes do split and link up again during cell division, but it is a random process (same old theme, mix up the genes). Imagine you have a piece of wood that is six feet long and you are going to cut it into two pieces with your eyes closed. If you paint two spots on the wood, one blue and the other red and the spots are five feet apart, the chances are that when you wildly swing your axe to cut the wood in half, the red spot will be on one piece and the blue on another. Repeat the process, however, with the red and blue spot six inches from each other and the chances that both will remain on the one piece of wood after it has been severed are very high. Immunoregulatory genes that look after such things as non-reaction to self are very close (in the geographical sense) to genes that code for HLA antigens. Hence, if you see a red spot, chances are that a blue spot is nearby.

A boy with diabetes, who also displays the DR3 DR4 combination, will very likely have a brother who also carries DR3 DR4 antigens on his cells and who may also be vulnerable to diabetes. With that suspicion, can we diagnose his disease early, well before most of his pancreas beta cells have been destroyed?

Glucagon is a hormone that stimulates the release of insulin from the pancreas into the bloodstream. A healthy pancreas will respond immediately to an injection of the hormone with the release of a specific amount of insulin. This normal response can be quantified, hence an abnormally low output of insulin would suggest that the pancreas is in trouble, though a long way as yet from clinical diabetes. If you follow the siblings of diabetic children or even their parents for ten years, those who have the same HLA profile as the family member with diabetes have an almost 100 per cent chance of developing the disease. Hence our interest in early diagnosis.

To recapitulate, some of us inherit a set of genes that do not establish the normal control mechanisms that stop attacks on self with the precision of another (obviously preferable) set of genes inherited by other individuals. As a result, some of us walk through life on a biological tightrope. But what things tend to disturb our precarious balance?

For the person with less than perfect immunoregulation the known environmental hazards are stress, drugs and infections, especially viral infections. The defect may be spontaneous or it may be triggered by some mechanisms currently unknown to us.

Psychological stress, especially when coping mechanisms cannot be generated can quite drastically disturb immunological function.

What about the ability of drugs to disturb immune control? All biological reactions can be translated into biochemical events in which soluble molecules move around the microenvironment arranging various sophisticated reactions. When you swallow that capsule, grimace at that injection or watch some therapeutic marvel dripping into your veins, you face a calculated risk associated with adding potent chemicals to a delicately balanced system.

Many drugs are wonderfully effective and safe for most of the population, yet they cause a lot of problems for people who live on an immunological tightrope. Antibiotics, drugs for controlling blood pressure, chemicals that make you pass a lot of urine, agents that control the rhythm of your heart etc., in fact more than one hundred commonly used drugs, can trigger off an autoimmune reaction in the susceptible individual.

What about infections? Viruses are the main culprits here, and we have yet to learn a great deal about how they damage self-control mechanisms. We know viruses can disturb the best of immune systems (e.g., in the case of AIDS) but less spectacular derangements occur with herpes viruses such as the one that causes mononucleosis and there are a number of other viruses that we think may be involved with specific diseases.

A nasty little virus called Coxsackie is a strong candidate for diabetes. There are at least two non-mutually exclusive possibilities here. A virus could decide that the beta cells of the pancreas would make the ideal home. Once ensconced, the virus may or may not damage its chosen residence. If viruses did damage the beta cells, their appearance could be so distorted that they may look 'foreign', that is, have membrane profiles different from those displayed on normal cells. In such circumstances immune cells may swoop on what they now perceive to be foreignness and may cause more harm than good by destroying not only the virus but the beta cells as well. The weaker our immunological self-control, the more likely we are to attack altered self. The alternative explanation involves viruses disturbing T cells directly, with the result that they behave inappropriately and attack self. Probably both these things happen simultaneously on many occasions.

With that background information, let us look at some of the autoimmune diseases themselves.

I should point out that these diseases are essentially those of women. For most of the conditions we will discuss, doctors see ten women with the problem for every male. It is true that men are worse affected than women, but fewer get these diseases. Why? The female immunologists of my acquaintance claim that men with such imperfections do not even make it out of the uterus to put up a fight. There may be a measure of truth in that but sex hormones do play an important role in setting up the regulation of the immune system.

Although we talk of 'this' and 'that' system within the body as if they

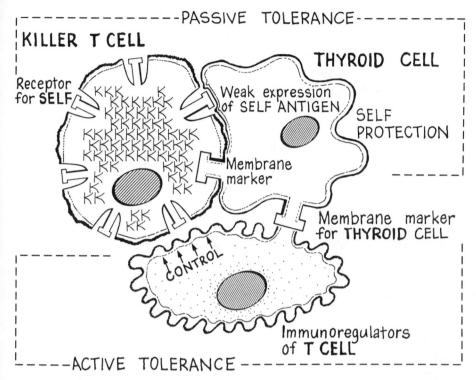

were independent if nicely integrated modules, in the real living body integration is so complete and the interdependence so profound that in reality there is just a functioning total system. We do not understand how, but an excess of male sex hormones (testosterones) over female sex hormones (particularly estrogens) tends to play a role in perfecting immunoregulation. Little female mice get an autoimmune disease seldom seen in their male litter mates. Giving girls testosterone from birth prevents them from developing the disease. (Of course, it also stops them from being girls.)

The diseases we call autoimmune fall into two big clusters. In one group of diseases specific organs tend to be targeted. Diabetes is obviously an example of that. In the other group, the problems are largely caused by immunological damage to blood vessels. Tissues relying on blood from the damaged vessels are themselves damaged.

The first group tends to occur in women and often there is a family history of this sort of disease among other females in the family. The victims have HLA profiles that suggest that their disease is caused by an immunogenetic deficiency that allows an autoimmune attack to occur. For reasons that are quite unknown, such cases frequently occur in women who have premature greying of the hair and often have small spots of depigmentation in their skin called vitiligo. Here are a few case reports to show you the range of these target orientated attacks.

One day I was observing a women screaming at a child of about four, obviously overreacting to the fact that the child's icecream had obeyed the laws of physics and a temperature of 104 °F, and had rapidly slid down the child to find the floor. As I looked at the woman I realised her hands were trembling seriously, she was in a lather of perspiration and she had very protruding eyes that looked as if they wanted to pop right out of her head. As I walked closer the diagnosis was clinched. A telltale swelling in the neck told all. The woman had an enlarged and overactive thyroid gland that was pouring forth the hormone thyroxine that drives so many of the body's metabolic processes. Too much and we tremble, we lose emotional control, we develop diarrhoea, changes in our hair and nails, disturbances of periods, severe weight loss, a racing heart and many other symptoms.

Unhesitatingly, but I hope politely, I asked the women if she knew she had a serious problem with her thyroid gland. For a moment I thought I might have a serious problem, so horrible was the stare she gave me, but she calmed down and told me that she had not sought medical help for her problem. I arranged for her to visit my professor the following week and indeed, the woman benefited significantly from the urgent treatment she was given.

What I did not realise at the time was that, in that unfortunate thyroid of hers, T and B cells had congregated and were literally destroying the gland. Some of the antibodies she was producing, directed against the cells of her thyroid gland actually stimulated them to release more and more hormone. The thyroid is a favorite target for autoimmunity when T cell regulation goes astray.

One of my favorite patients has diabetes and another autoimmune disease. At the age of twenty-nine, she was referred by her doctor because of increasingly frequent episodes of muscular weakness. She runs a nursery and has the soft, caring personality one so often finds in people who work with trees, flowers and plants.

Ellen was a strong girl, although not big, and was used to lifting plants around her nursery and unloading bags of fertiliser and the like. For the few months before she consulted me she had noticed that walking up a flight of stairs made her legs feel extremely weak. She could unload the first two bags of fertiliser from a delivery truck but then strangely each subsequent bag got heavier and heavier until she could not move her arms at all. After some rest, she would recover. She also complained that she was having trouble with her eyes. When reading for any length of time she would develop double vision.

On asking her to open and close her hands repeatedly one could quickly see how soon she tired and we immediately suspected that she suffered from myasthenia (muscle weakness) gravis (severe). Our investigations supported the diagnosis and we rushed her into hospital and had our best surgeons open her chest to remove her thymus gland. Remove her thymus gland? The soul of her immune system? Yes, I know it sounds shocking, but let me explain.

Myasthenia gravis is perhaps the most fascinating of all the autoimmune diseases (and can be one of the most serious). To understand it you have to know how nerves tell muscles to move. Please tell your left hand to form a fist right now. From the time your mind said 'okay' to my request and the time your hand formed a fist was but a fraction of a second. From your cerebral cortex a message sped at incredible speed down the nerves in your spinal column to move out to and then down the nerves in your arms to your hand.

When the electrical message carried by your nerves got to the muscle, however, a change occurred. Between the end of the nerve and the trigger point on the muscle which must be activated for it to move, there is a gap. Across that space the message from the nerve telling your hand to move will be carried, not in the form of electricity, but in the form of a chemical. It is like a breathless runner arriving at the edge of a river bank and begging a man to row him across to the opposite side so that he can deliver a message to a person waiting there. The chemical reaction is almost as quick as the electrical one, however. The chemical races across the gap and binds to the trigger point on the muscle, which is stimulated by this chemical. The substance in question for most muscles is called acetylcholine (ACH) and the trigger point in question on our muscle is called, reasonably enough, the receptor for ACH.

Myasthenia occurs when we make an immunological attack on that receptor, which becomes covered in antibodies. The result is that it is very difficult for the ACH to get its message through.

We all get tired muscles if we work them continuously but after just a few contractions people with myasthenia gravis cannot supply sufficient amounts of acetylcholine to break through the antibody barrier and stimulate the muscles. Should the receptors that are being blocked be on muscles involved in making the chest wall move, without the help of mechanical respirators, patients could die.

Why remove the thymus? Thousands of years ago, the thymus had two jobs; the production of T cells, of course, but also the production of a hormone we no longer appear to need that actually facilitated neuro-muscular transmission. To produce the hormone, the thymus had in its tissues a few isolated muscle cells with receptors for acetylcholine. These odd muscle cells are still to be found in the human thymus.

In patients with myasthenia gravis, within their thymus gland T cells suddenly attack those muscle cells as if they were foreign and it appears that the specific antigen that irritates them is the receptor for the neurotransmitter. It would not matter so much if the attack stayed in the thymus gland which, as we have discussed before, is not a very important organ in adult life, but the T and B cells which we can see congregating in the thymus in this disease, leave this organ and go out to the peripheral muscles and attack important receptors. The dissemination of these auto-aggressive cells from the thymus can be minimised by surgically removing the thymus. We try to do this as early as possible in the disease.

Other diseases that fall into the same mechanistic category, that is, a deliberate immunological attack on a specific tissue, include pernicious anemia, where an antibody is formed that blocks the ability of an intestinal hormonal-like agent known as 'intrinsic factor' to absorb vitamin B12. This vitamin is essential for the production of red blood cells and the health of our nervous system. In other diseases the ovaries, the testes, the parathyroid glands that control calcium metabolism, our red blood cells and our platelets can all be attacked and seriously damaged.

There is a second large cluster of diseases, however, where an immune system's deranged behaviour causes damage in another way. The proto-type of such diseases is systemic lupus erythematosus, abbreviated by doctors and patients alike to SLE. Thousands of people suffer from this disease which has, as its basis, damage to blood vessels.

Mrs L. was a thirty-five-year-old married mother of two healthy children when she returned from a two-week holiday in Jamaica feeling decidedly unwell with painful joints, a moderate fever, a feeling of overwhelming doom and a strange rash on her face. She thought at first that she had been suffering from sunburn but soon realised that this was different. From one cheek to the other a red scaly rash had appeared which narrowed to bridge her nose in butterfly-like fashion. Her family doctor recognised the characteristic rash of SLE and she was sent to us for investigation. We controlled her disease but could not cure her; she remains only moderately well.

What had happened to Mrs L? A T cell malfunction had been triggered, as so often happens in these cases, by exposure to ultraviolet light (which can disturb less than perfect immunoregulatory cells). As a result she had begun to make antibodies to her own tissues. In the case of SLE the target seems harmless enough. Every day we constantly regenerate lost cells, that part of us which died yesterday, and the debris is usually cleared from our system by an inhouse garbage collecting organisation featuring scavenger cells that can literally eat tissue debris. The system is mainly focussed in the liver and spleen.

Poor Mrs L's lymphocytes were making antibodies to the naked nuclei of cells that had died and were being removed. These antinuclear antibodies were being produced in great quantities. As the garbage system was trying to remove the nuclear material, the antibodies bound themselves to these proteins, forming big complexes that the scavenger cells found hard to deal with. As a result some complexes were not cleared rapidly enough from blood vessels. The complexes were then becoming trapped in certain sites in her body, usually tiny blood vessels, and the immune response that followed featured a lot of damage to the blood vessels that were unfortunate enough to be clogged with these complexes. The blood vessels became inflamed, lost their patency and a number of tissues suffered.

SLE primarily affects skin, joints, the central nervous system and the kidneys. The last are particularly vulnerable. Why people suddenly start making antibodies to self debris is not clear but genetic and environmental factors (in this case sunlight) are very important. Many diseases feature this kind of pathology rather than the organ-orientated approach seen with, for example, thyroid disease. Rheumatoid arthritis is another classical example.

With ageing there is a natural tendency for self-control to diminish so that autoimmune diseases and phenomena may appear late in life when the integrity of our very definitely finite T cell system starts to wane. Fortunately, there is a lot we can do for many of these problems, but we cannot cure them. This subject then is a distressing one providing yet another example of how the development of ever more sophisticated weaponry for defense leaves the defenders in great danger if the forces they control turn inwards. Wasn't it poor Guillotin who lost his head at the knife of his most famous invention?

9 | The chronic fatigue syndrome: an immunological mystery disease

FOR immunology, and indeed most medical disciplines, the truism 'the more you know, the more you realise how much you don't know' is undoubtedly accurate. That is not to say that this truism is perceived as such by the majority of physicians. If anything, the story that follows would suggest the opposite. The case histories that follow illustrate how patients with unusual symptoms that currently defy explanation are too easily considered to be hypochondriacs, victims of a neurosis.

Carol is twenty-eight and introduced herself to me as a 'debilitated airline stewardess'. She had led a normal life until the age of twenty-four when happiness and a bright future turned to despair in a matter of months.

Carol flew international routes for a wellknown airline and had been doing so since she was nineteen. She was pretty, popular and an excellent athlete. Sure, she would get tired after eight hours with 400 people in a jumbo jet, but she recovered quickly and enjoyed her stopovers. She had a multitude of interests which she was able to accommodate despite her hectic jetting around the globe.

Her problems started on a flight to London. She remembers leaving New York in perfect health but was feeling decidedly unwell three hours into the flight. At this point she had a headache, a sore throat and some muscle aches. She was able to work but she remembers thinking to herself, 'I am in for a bad dose of the flu.' By the time she arrived in London, all her symptoms were worse and she was sure she had a temperature. She went back to her hotel and by 7 am was in bed, hoping that six hours of sleep would see the virus spent and her good health returned to her.

190

She fell into a deep sleep and woke at 5 pm considerably worse. Her nightdress was soaked from perspiration and she was experiencing a shaking chill. Never could she recall having a throat as sore as the one she awoke to; never had she felt so wretched. Realising that she was unusually sick she called for the hotel doctor who came promptly, examined her carefully and confirmed that indeed she had a high temperature. He told her that almost certainly she was suffering from glandular fever, alternatively referred to as infectious mononucleosis. He informed her that the very severe pharyngitis she was experiencing was typical of this particular viral infection. Aspirin and antibiotics were prescribed, the first for the fever and pain, the second to ward off any secondary bacterial complications. Blood tests were ordered for the following day to confirm his diagnosis. In the meantime she was to drink a lot of fluid and rest completely. Carol had no choice but to follow the latter advice for, as she recalled, she felt utterly exhausted.

After four days in her hotel bed she felt considerably improved. Though she still felt weak the sore throat and fever had all but gone. She arranged to fly home (as a passenger; she was not well enough to work) and remembers being somewhat uneasy when her English physician told her as she departed that all her blood tests had been negative, i.e., he had been unable to confirm a diagnosis of glandular fever. Despite this, he remained confident that 'mono' was the cause of her problems and that in six weeks she would be her old self again.

We have discussed the common problem known as infectious mononucleosis already. This disease is caused by a virus from the herpes family that invades almost 100 per cent of us at some time in our lives, usually before the age of twenty-five. For reasons that are not altogether clear, infections in childhood, especially before the age of six, rarely result in any significant symptoms. When one is infected with the virus it can be found in saliva and therefore can be spread as a droplet infection and move easily into bodies that come close to those that are infected. A cough or a sneeze can discharge thousands of viral particles into the air around us. It is particularly well transmitted by kissing, hence it is frequently, if somewhat romantically, described at the 'kissing disease'.

The particular virus involved is called the Epstein-Barr virus after its discoverers. It is unique in that, in addition to invading our throats and liver cells, it also takes up residence in our B cells. Once it invades these antibody-producing cells the only way to get rid of it is to kill those infected B cells. This our T cells eventually manage to do. As most B cells live in our lymph glands, the battle between the EB virus and our T cells is fought out in these glands that become swollen and tender, hence the alternative name of 'glandular fever'.

For a period that varies from one individual to another, the immune

192 I THE BODY AT WAR

system is disturbed by an infection with the 'mono' virus and inappropriate immunological reactions can take place. For example, patients often develop allergies for the first time and experience autoimmune disorders during that phase of the illness which occurs before the T cells manage to kill the virus. A number of patients may remain ill for months as they battle the virus. They have a long-drawn-out, i.e., continuous, infection. Other patients infected with an equal dose of the same virus don't even know that they have met up with such a challenge, so efficiently does their immune system handle the invasion. The range of scenarios observed following an infection by the EB virus is determined by the variety of genetic programs available to direct, more or less efficiently, the immunological attack against the virus. The potency of the virus is constant, the host response is variable. The 'mono' we have been discussing is not what troubled Carol, but as EBV will become a central player in our mystery disease, the previous explanation was necessary.

On returning to New York, Carol saw her own doctor who felt that her English physician was most likely correct and ordered her to bed for two further weeks of complete rest. A good patient, she did as she was told and got her reward. After two weeks she felt 95 per cent better and was ready to return to work. Further blood tests had not shown the presence of antibody to the EB virus so the diagnosis of infectious mononucleosis seemed unsustainable. Her physician told her that her problem, now almost resolved, must have been caused by something similar to the EB virus.

At her doctor's insistence, Carol took a further ten day's rest before she returned to work, ready to get on with her life. Shortly thereafter, however, our mysterious disease struck in full force.

Two months into her normal routine, Carol would have said she was still struggling slightly to regain full health, being about 85 per cent of her former energetic self. Then, on one easily remembered morning, she awoke, only to find that overnight her body had departed and a new one had been slipped into her bed.

Her new body was that of a very old woman, she thought. It protested that it did not want to move; it was exhausted. More than that, it ached from head to toe. She could feel each muscle protesting even as she lay immobile in the bed. Many of the muscles felt tender to her touch. With the maximum amount of willpower she dragged her new self to the bathroom, then collapsed back on her bed, utterly exhausted from this effort. She had been tired before but never had she felt anything approaching this sensation. Her head was pounding and she recalls how confused she was. Certainly she could not work in this condition and this was worrisome as she had an uneasy feeling that she was meant to work that day. Try as she might, however, she could not bring her mind to focus on her timetable. As she tried to analyse her working movements over the past week she felt herself incapable of the mental agility required. Carol called her airline, found that she was indeed due to fly to Frankfurt, apologised, said she was sick and withdrew her services, much to the chagrin of the rostering clerk.

When her doctor arrived she told him how she felt and promptly burst into a bout of uncontrollable crying. She remembers the sobbing that accompanied an overwhelming feeling of depression. The doctor, the same caring physician she had consulted earlier on her return from England, admitted that he was confused. He could find nothing abnormal on examination of his patient and told Carol so. 'You might be coming down with another virus, Carol, or this could be a flare-up of your 'mono'; that can happen, you know. In any case stay in bed, rest and I am sure it will either declare itself or pass off quickly and you can get back to work.' Carol has not returned to work and it is now four years since the start of her problem.

What followed for Carol can only be imagined in the context of a nightmare. This new body of hers was out to torture her. She had days when some of her exhaustion lifted but if she tried to do even the simplest task for herself she would experience three days of such extreme fatigue that she could not force herself to walk across a room.

Carol returned to her parents' home where sympathy was forthcoming. As the months rolled by, however, sympathy gave way to puzzlement and frustration set in for patient and family alike. Her own physician performed a battery of tests and nothing abnormal turned up in any of the high-technology screening programs called upon to analyse her blood.

As the agony continued, some major symptoms were most consistent: headaches that were not typical for either tension or migraine blighted her every morning, the mental confusion and emotional lability that descended on her 'like a veil being placed over my mind' continued and even worsened. This once energetic and resourceful young woman was but a shadow of her former self. In addition to these two constant symptoms, her extreme fatigue and muscle aches continued.

She noted other things about herself. Sometimes eating made her fatigue worse and her daily nightmare did not leave her in sleep. She was attacked almost nightly by horrifying meaningless nightmares, most notable for the vivid colours featured. She often found her muscles jerking and twitching uncontrollably when she tried to move them.

Of course she was referred to a consultant physician for help. The first considered that her increased fatigue after eating was due to low blood sugar levels, a not uncommon problem associated with an overenthusiastic release of insulin after sugar is ingested. The usual dietary manipulations that help patients with this problem did not, however, help Carol. After that, many physicians tackled her problem, all remaining puzzled and unhelpful in the face of her constellation of symptoms. The third consultant, in what was to be a series of sixteen, looked at his totally unrewarding test results, looked at Carol and told her calmly and confidently that she was suffering from a psychological rather than an organic problem. She was troubled by a severe neurosis; urgent psychiatric help was essential.

She dutifully accepted the advice and consulted a psychiatrist, an older man with a down-to-earth disposition. After a number hours of discussion and examination he told an anxious patient and her desperate parents that he could find nothing untoward in her personality that wasn't entirely explained by the frustration of her situation. As this did not seem to be of much help to Carol, it was decided that a second and younger psychiatrist should be consulted. This was done and he came to exactly the opposite opinion. This man seized on the fact that just before Carol's well-remembered trip to London when she first became ill she had terminated a romance; this, he declared, was the undoubted cause of her problem.

When Carol pointed out that it was she who had called off the affair and that indeed she had been relieved to be out of an unsatisfactory situation, her explanation fell on Freudian ears that saw a plethora of subconscious reasons for her psychosomatic disorder. Urged on by her parents, Carol entered into therapy with this man. After six months, however, both patient and doctor were frustrated at any lack of progress and agreed to part company.

Unfortunately her psychotherapy failed Carol in two ways. Not only did it not help her but indeed it harmed her. Her employer, friends and even her family were instantly convinced that psychotherapy meant that hers was a real psychiatric disease. Bizarre symptoms in the face of normal blood tests are so easily dismissed as neurosis.

After two years of all this, Carol was spiritually alone, severely depressed, weak, confused and, pathetic. Her once vital smile and twinkling eyes had been replaced by a despondent, lifeless stare. Some of the doctors she consulted along her painful journey were humble enough to discuss their ignorance and the possibility that this was a strange but definite disease. What were they to make of a patient whose muscles looked normal (even under the microscope), were not wasted, as occurs in patients with polio, responded normally to electric stimulation, yet would not allow Carol to walk around the block without extracting a penalty of three days' absolute rest in bed before letting her move again?

Carol was certainly not the first patient I had seen with this problem; far from it. Two hundred or so similar patients and approximately fifteen years earlier I had been consulted by an airline pilot (a coincidence, I know, but I am not suggesting that flying is any way linked to this problem). He could no longer fly his jumbo jet, not only because he was too weak but because he could no longer make the accurate and swift decisions needed for his profession. He told me a tale similar in many ways to that told by Carol but his problem was less severe. His troubles had started with a well-documented attack of glandular fever. He developed quite readily detectable antibodies to the Epstein-Barr virus during his flulike illness.

Now, as many of you will know from recent publicity all around the world, the fatigue syndrome we are discussing is far from rare. Depending on the part of the world in which you live it is variously referred to as the Iceland syndrome, Royal Free disease, epidemic neuromyasthenia, chronic EBV syndrome, myalgic encephalomyelitis (ME), post-infection fatigue syndrome or the term that we will use throughout this chapter, the chronic fatigue syndrome (CFS). I prefer the last title as it doesn't pretend that we know more than we do. To put our knowledge about CFS into historical perspective let us look at how this disease, whatever one may call it, first came to medical attention.

In London in 1955, trouble was brewing (incubating might be a better word) at one of that city's great teaching hospitals, the Royal Free. Ancient, admirable and academic, this hospital had much to be proud of. One of the finest liver units in the world had been established there and the attending physicians read like a *Who's Who* of UK medicine. On 13 July, two of the staff, one doctor, one nurse, reported to the appropriate hospital clinic with a puzzling and similar condition. They were admitted to the hospital for investigation. Over the next two weeks seventy more of the staff came down with the same illness and were also admitted. While all the staff were greatly concerned at these developments, panic was absent for, after all, this was a hospital whose staff had been dealing with the dangerous polio epidemic for years. As hospital officials could not be certain what was happening to their staff it seemed prudent to close the hospital; in any case, staff were now in short supply. On 25 July this great hospital closed its doors and did not open them until October. During that time 292 members of the staff were seen with similar symptoms and 255 were admitted. Obviously an epidemic of something was occurring, but what?

The patients all had similar symptoms, though the severity and mixture of symptoms varied. Headaches, emotional lability, extreme tiredness, pain in the back, neck and often one limb, dizziness, troublesome blurring of vision and swollen lymph glands were all common. Most worrying were clear signs that the major nerves running inside the head were not functioning normally. Twenty per cent had paralysis of the muscles of their face, many had difficulty swallowing, muscle spasms, double vision and sensory disturbances.

Most of the staff recovered fairly quickly but the major persistent problem, noted time and time again, was extreme muscle fatigue. No infectious agent was found that could explain the epidemic but it was presumed that some new agent, probably a virus, had swept through the hospital and that this virus had a specific predilection for muscle and the nervous system. For some of the staff of the Royal Free Hospital the disease did not disappear rapidly but persisted for many weeks, months and for a small number, indefinitely. With no causative agent found it was quite understandable that the problem was called, for want of anything more scientific, 'Royal Free disease'.

What the physicians struggling with the problem at the Royal Free Hospital did not know was that in February of that year an outbreak of a very similar disease had occurred in three areas in north west London. To the Royal Free symptoms were added a very rapid pulse rate and vivid technicolor nightmares. Apart from these additional symptoms the problems described by these patients were identical to those given by the staff of the Royal Free Hospital.

With the publication in 1957 of the Royal Free story in medical literature, reports started to come in from all around the world describing similar outbreaks. For example in February 1955, at the time north west London was experiencing this problem, a similar outbreak occurred in a hospital in Durban, South Africa.

Investigators interested in this problem have now agreed that the first outbreak of the 'Royal Free disease' occurred in the Los Angeles County General Hospital in 1934. More than thirty-five outbreaks have been recorded around the world with major ones occurring in Iceland in 1948, Adelaide, South Australia in 1949 and in numerous other places, suggesting that this is not a geographically restricted problem.

In the late 1960s scientists were becoming interested in the problem of Royal Free disease when a 'disastrous advance' occurred. Just as investigators proposed the name myalgic (painful muscles) encephalomyelitis (inflammation of brain and nerves), usually abbreviated to ME, as a satisfactory name for the disorder, two psychologists unwittingly but arrogantly brought research into this disease to an abrupt halt.

The two investigators in question had recently experienced a major triumph and were looking for a follow-up. They had been called in to examine an epidemic of painful muscle spasm among young ladies attending an all-girls' school in England.

Interested, indeed expert in mass hysteria, they were soon able to attribute the painful spasms of the hands and the tingling of the lips felt by the girls to overbreathing; mass hysteria leading to epidemic panic and hyperventilation. Increasing one's rate of breathing when it is not demanded by physical activity soon results in too much carbon dioxide being released from the body. The acid content of blood and tissues falls, nerves become highly irritable and spasm results.

The two doctors asked the Royal Free Hospital for permission to review the records of those patients affected during the famous epidemic. The hypothesis they wished to test argued that those affected would be found to be predisposed to psychoneuroses. In 1970 they published their opinion that the Royal Free epidemic was indeed a marvellous example of mass hysteria and that similar outbreaks in the world would be similarly explained. The confidence of these psychologists was hardly justified when one considers that they did not see the patients and saw no inconsistency associated with the fact that 79 per cent of the patients had swollen lymph glands, 89 per cent had a fever, 45 per cent had paralysis of their eye muscles and 19 per cent were unable to move their facial muscles; all signs that are hard to produce hysterically.

The damage was done, however, and the media seized upon this sensational explanation as an example of how improved medical sophistication allowed modern doctors to understand that personality disorders, not new organic diseases, would provide the new syndromes.

The *Sunday Times* in London and no less a medical authority than *Time* magazine accepted without question the hysteria explanation and in so doing added enormously to the suffering of many thousands of far-from-hysterical individuals afflicted with the chronic fatigue syndrome. The public, many of the patients themselves, and countless numbers of physicians, uncomfortable with their inability to understand the disease in organic terms, accepted the hysteria explanation and the syndrome became almost invariably regarded as a neurosis.

The best scientists are similar to the best detectives. They can't throw away major clues just because they distort some preconceived suspicion. Our psychologists surely should have couched their conclusions on a bed of reservations, admitting that there were some clues that didn't fit their hypothesis. Surely their unequivocal diagnosis of mass hysteria should have been more restrained, as the medical records of many of the patients detailed that it was necessary to feed them via a rubber tube inserted into their stomach, so severe was the paralysis of muscles needed to swallow.

Physicians who deal with patients suffering chronic illnesses know, if they are at all perceptive, that psychological problems develop as a result of the frustrations of living with poor health. Often such a situation challenges the physician to use both his art and his science to dissect the functional away from the organic. Both elements of the disease process demand treatment, but different treatment. It is in no way surprising that many, indeed most patients with a chronic fatigue syndrome have some psychological turmoil increasing the misery orchestrated by their basic disease.

The prominence of symptoms such as emotional lability, depression, impaired memory and powers of concentration is consistent. They are, in my opinion, caused by the disease itself and thus do not represent the secondary psychological problems discussed above.

To summarise to this point. Chronic fatigue syndromes have been described since 1934. It is perfectly reasonable to presume that they have occurred for much longer but were submerged in a sea of serious life-threatening diseases. Patients with CFS may have developed their disability sequelae of either flulike illness that swept through their community (an epidemic) or a disease-causing event that selected them from among the healthy majority (endemic form). In the former case it is most reasonable to presume that an as yet unidentified infectious agent (virus?) is responsible. For those with long-term complications, in contra-distinction to the majority who recovered quickly, an inherent defect compromising their attack on the causal agent seems likely. In the latter situation a less virulent form of the same agent, ineffectual in its attempts to damage the majority, might have settled for a host less able to resist this particular infection for genetic reasons. Alternatively, we could be discussing two quite separate diseases.

In both suggested scenarios, a host defect is forwarded as a predis-posing factor for the development of CFS. What could this factor be? A genetic defect downgrading the efficiency of a response to infection should translate into an immunological defect, and this suggestion has now been established as fact. The reproduceable demonstration of T-cell abnormalities in patients with CFS is the reason we are discussing this disease.

At the time of this writing, we are far from a complete understanding of the molecular events that ultimately produce the symptoms that so devastate our patients but there is no longer any doubt that the syndrome we are discussing is primarily organic, not psychological. Thousands of patients previously labelled as neurotic have been vindicated. Unfortu-nately continued widespread ignorance of the condition perpetuates psychological harrassment for many.

Patients with classical symptoms of CFS almost always have reduced numbers of immunoregulatory cells in their blood. The number of inducer or alarm-sounding T cells is also often reduced. Another almost universal finding from my unit's research has been anergy: patients with CFS cannot respond satisfactorily to antigens injected into their skin. So consistent are these abnormalities that when they are coupled to specific symptoms they allow us to make a positive diagnosis, rather than one that results from exclusion of other problems.

The concept of a genetic defect that results in a less-than-ideal performance by immunoregulatory cells allows us to better understand an increasingly appreciated fact about CFS.

In the endemic form, many different foreign (non-self) agents appear to be capable of triggering CFS. This is the reason why I don't like the term 'post-infection fatigue syndrome'. CFS can be triggered by foreign proteins incapable of causing an infection. This is most commonly observed following the administration of a vaccine or antigen to boost the immune response.

Harry at thirty-six was thoroughly enjoying his family and work as the supervisor of a national park when CFS struck. Typical of people who spend their life protecting nature, Harry was softly spoken, ruggedly healthy and at peace with himself and the world around him. One day he was cleaning an area in his forest that had been polluted by some visitors. They had left behind cans and bottles to prove how little they had appreciated the beauty that they had come to explore. While pulling a can from the soil Harry cut his finger, not badly but possibly, he thought, a stitch would be needed. He drove to the local community hospital where the doctor considered a bandage would suffice but ordered a precautionary tetanus toxoid booster. Harry had not had such a shot for ten years and the advice was therefore appropriate. Twelve hours after his tetanus shot Harry was in trouble. He had developed a high fever, shaking chills and and a severe headache. He retreated to his bed. There was no reaction at the site of the tetanus shot, excluding an extremely vigorous immune reaction to the tetanus antigen itself as the cause of the problem. Such reactions do occur if one has too many tetanus shots too frequently.

Harry did not improve for three days and then made a partial recovery. He returned to work after a week but felt totally exhausted. His weariness persisted. Three years later Harry has not returned to his forest. For him to walk around his house is to be sentenced to six hours in bed to recuperate. He is still racked with headaches and a mental fuzziness that impairs his memory and concentration. I have observed this type of reaction many times and yet we know that for the vast majority, a tetanus shot is a harmless, indeed life-preserving stimulus to our immune system. A tetanus shot does not cause CFS but it can trigger a chain of events, as yet poorly understood, that may lead to CFS.

In the United Kingdom the most common triggers for CFS are enteroviruses. These are a family of tiny viruses that like to live in our intestinal tract (hence 'entero' meaning enteric or bowel). It may be of considerable significance that the particular enterovirus associated with CFS in the UK, the Coxsackie virus, is a close relative of the demons that cause polio. Coxsackie viruses were discovered forty years ago in the feces of two children suspected of having polio. We now know that there are seventy-one members of the enterovirus family which include not only the polio-producing viruses and the Coxsackie family but also the ECHO viruses that are responsible for a number of diseases. All multiply within the intestinal tract.

Coxsackie is a delightful little village on the banks of the Hudson

River in New York State. The local residents regard with some chagrin the fact that their main claim to fame is that it was from their residents that the nasty enteroviruses we are discussing were first isolated.

In experimental animals and humans there is no doubt that Coxsackie virus can damage both muscles and nervous tissue. These are highly infectious viruses and if one member of the family becomes infected there is a 76 per cent chance that other members will also become infected. Recent evidence suggests that in genetically programmed individuals a particular Coxsackie virus can trigger off the immunological attack on the pancreas that may cause juvenile onset diabetes.

In the United States, the Epstein-Barr virus that may cause glandular fever and precipitate a number of cancers has long been considered a major trigger for CFS. No matter which side of the Atlantic we review, no matter which agent acts as a trigger (Coxsackie, tetanus, parasites, EBV, etc.) the syndrome is identical.

Logic demands that we broaden the hypothesis that we discussed earlier. A unique virus may cause epidemic CFS but any number of foreign proteins (including a less virulent form of the epidemic-producing virus), upon entering a host with a specific defect in his immune system, can produce the same syndrome.

Most recently a new candidate has appeared that might trigger CFS. This is a herpes virus (they are always bad news) called HBLV; H for human, B for B cells where it likes to live, L for lymphocyte and V for virus. American investigators found antibodies to this virus in many of their CFS patients. We looked at our patients and found the same thing. The problem is that it is now clear that infection with this virus is ubiquitous; most of our control subjects have also been infected at one time or another. Thus HBLV may be another potential trigger for endemic CFS but it is not the sole cause, as it does not produce the syndrome in the majority of people that it infects.

In the last two years a series of definite abnormalities have been discovered in patients with CFS. With this new and tantalising data, scientists have before them a complicated jigsaw puzzle with 50 per cent of the pieces available. While the outline of the biological design is just visible, there is enough of a pattern to allow one to generate a more informed series of testable hypotheses. What are these new data?

The symptoms of patients with CFS suggest that they have a problem that has developed within their muscles. They ache and they feel weak. Such symptoms could arise in people with perfectly normal muscles if the part of the brain normally charged with interpreting signals coming from muscles is itself defective. In CFS, however, it is far more likely that the muscles themselves have been damaged by the disease. Then the weakness and pain messages being received by the brain are clearly and accurately interpreted as a desire on the part of the muscles not to move.

Is there evidence for muscle damage?

Magnetic resonance imaging (MRI) is a technological breakthrough of major importance. As X-ray techniques gave way to computer assisted imaging (CAT scans), so they in turn will yield to MRI. Just as powerful satellite cameras can now image from space the chess moves being made by a pair of old men relaxing in a park, our medical cameras can now actually look at molecular events occurring in our bodies. Muscles, for example are made up of fibres, which in turn are made up of fibrils, which are made up of proteins, which are made up of atoms, which are made up of electrons and neutrons and protons moving around each other in the most disciplined dance in all biology. MRI allows us to look at these events in a given tissue and compare the molecular events seen in diseased tissue with those observed in healthy tissue. Using this technology, reports are reaching us of distinct biochemical abnormalities within the muscles of people with CFS.

Electronmicroscopic examination of muscle biopsies reveal subtle but definite changes in muscle fibres and their cells. Suddenly the old claim of many physicians that there is nothing wrong with the muscles of patients with CFS falls into perspective. Previous investigators have not used techniques capable of finding the subtle defects that are now observable. As it is obviously more difficult to biopsy brain than muscle tissue we must presume at the moment that similar biochemical events are affecting central nervous function.

What causes the biochemical defects that lead to the disturbance of function? There are a number of possibilities, none mutually exclusive. One possibility would involve the persistence in an affected tissue of inadequately cleared particles of the triggering agent that would directly interfere with muscle enzymes or other vital biochemicals needed for muscle function. Another would see those particles as stimulators of a chronic immunological attack that would damage the normal 'innocent bystander' tissue. Yet another mechanism would have genetic programs carried by viruses reprogram normal cells that would subsequently function abnormally. All these explanations immediately incriminate the immune system which should have dispatched any triggering agents to the immunological garbage heap within days of its entering our body.

Recent studies in the United Kingdom using modern genetic technology have discovered that at least some particles of Coxsackie viruses persist within the muscles of some patients with CFS. This certainly strengthens the argument of those who feel that partially degraded antigens are responsible for CFS.

Whether it will turn out to be significant for CFS or not, there is great interest in recent data which has confirmed the possibility that an unusual form of persistent viral infection may be responsible for a number of disease processes. We know that once herpes viruses enter our bodies, they never leave. For most of us, this is not a problem. They live quietly and harmlessly along nerve sheaths or in B cells without disturbing the function of a tissue or the cells they have invaded. This peaceful state of affairs has nothing to do with any inherent benignity on the part of the virus. Should the watchful eyes of our immune system falter, these viruses will seize the opportunity to multiply and invade. Shingles is the classical example of such a consequence.

What we are now realising is that viruses may enter a tissue or cell and change its *function*, while our immune system shows no interest. This is a new concept of infection. Doctors and lay people alike are used to the concept that organisms invade and damage a tissue as they multiply and release toxins, etc. The battle that follows, in which immunological forces produce their chemical warfare, temporarily adds to miseries of the invaded tissue and its owner. A climactic battle usually sees victory for our immune system, the invader is rejected and the innocent tissue that hosted the battle slowly repairs itself.

The ingenuity of viruses, however, now presents us with another scenario. In this version of infection a virus dives into a cell and inserts its genetic program into the cell's computer (the DNA of its nucleus), so changing the functional instructions of that cell. We now believe that some viruses may do this without interfering with the mechanisms that protect the outer wall of the cell. This second trick is essential if our immune system is to be fooled. Usually, when viruses invade cells, the fact is recognised by our immune system as components that are 'non-self' appear on a cell surface. T cells will destroy such cells and the viruses they contain.

In discussing CFS we are interested in the concept that some viruses, perhaps only in genetically susceptible people, cause disease not by destroying the cells they invade but by altering their specialised function. Subtle invasion of nerve and muscle cells in a manner that could destroy normal function without destroying the cells and evade partially compromised immunological surveillance mechanisms would explain the CFS mystery. Such a concept is hard to reconcile with the observation that non-viable proteins (e.g. tetanus) can trigger CFS.

We are investigating the theory that any number of antigens lodged in muscles and nervous tissue may be attacked chronically but suboptimally by a defective set of T cells. Normal tissue is damaged by the constantly high concentration of chemicals meant to be present in tissues for only a brief period. If you examine the side effects of interferon, a T-cell product normally released transiently in the course of an infection but now available for therapeutic purposes, the side effects associated with too high a dose are very similar to CFS.

This brings us to an immunological therapy that is potentially the most exciting breakthrough we have had in our attempts to help people with

CFS. Immunologists are currently fascinated by the beneficial effects of very large doses of gammaglobulin infused intravenously. Preparations of almost pure IgG extracted and concentrated from the blood of 3000 or more healthy humans are available commercially.

While the administration of this preparation to patients who can't make IgG is lifesaving, we have been excited by the discovery that many patients with autoimmune disease are markedly improved after very large doses of this preparation. Patients whose immune system has lost direction and is destroying their platelets or red cells, blocking nerve and muscle interactions, eating away at their joints, destroying their skin, etc., have been helped, sometimes dramatically, by an infusion of gammaglobulin.

We are far from certain how the pharmacological doses that we administer work their magic, but we are not short of theories. To me the most interesting observation concerns the improvement in regulatory T cell function that may follow these infusions. Large doses of IgG may well re-regulate a disordered T cell symptom.

In 1986, a friend of mine in New Jersey, told me that he had given a large dose of IgG to a patient with CFS and a remarkable improvement had followed. We speculated on the possible mechanisms. I decided to try this approach on a young man with a very severe form of the disease.

Jason was nineteen years old and devastated by a weakness that 'words cannot describe'. He was so weak that it could take him an hour to move from his living room to the bathroom. Such an effort would leave him so exhausted that he would need to spend five to six hours in his bed to recover to a point where he could sit up and converse with the rest of the family.

Two years earlier Jason had been set for a brilliant if unusual career. He was a champion surfboard rider and at the age of seventeen he had actually ranked third in the world. Day in, day out, he spent his time dancing on the tops and bottoms of waves. He was extremely fit.

Disaster struck Jason with a typical 'mono' like flu with fevers for a week, sore throat and swollen glands and the onset of a weakness that did not leave him. As the months passed, Jason became weaker and embarked on that all-too-familiar journey of frustration that so adds to the misery of CFS sufferers. Doctor after doctor was consulted to no avail.

Finally an eminent psychiatrist confidently told Jason and his frustrated parents that fear of the pressure of competition had produced a psychological cripple. This was his way of withdrawing with dignity from the pressures of the professional surfriding circuit on which he had been about to embark. They believed the consultant and fed antidepressant medicines to their now thoroughly depressed son. He did not improve.

We could find nothing abnormal on physical examination when Jason finally arrived at our clinic. I say 'finally' because twice he had missed appointments as he experienced the embarrassment of calling a taxi and then being unable to remember where the taxi was supposed to take him. Only when his parents, both of whom work, left written instructions did Jason make it to our clinic.

Jason was willing to try the IgG therapy and his response was most encouraging. In the week following a three-day infusion, he felt worse, if anything. His muscles ached and we could actually see the quivering as a myriad tiny contractions raced along muscle fibres. He had pains in his chest and a feeling of anxiety. Then, 'as if a devil had left my body', he awoke one morning feeling incredibly light; a sensation that his body was floating in a swimming pool swept over him. As he left his bed he felt energy for the first time in three years. Three months later Jason was tentatively challenging the waves and now a year later he feels he is ready for competition. I much enjoyed writing the follow-up letter to his psychiatrist.

We have now treated more than 80 patients with severe CFS with this therapy: 70 per cent have been significantly improved and we feel that 40 per cent are cured, though our confidence in that opinion will increase when a little more time has passed.

The path to scientific hell is paved with uncontrolled trials and anecdotes. I am cautiously optimistic that this therapy will result in a double breakthrough in our battle with the CFS problem. Firstly, we will help many patients recover, though it is already certain that not all respond; a fact that demands its own research. Secondly, it challenges immunologists to find out why IgG helps. If we can find the explanation we will surely be closer to understanding the basic cause of the disease.

It is possible that pooled gammaglobulin contains antibodies to a specific virus that is commonly experienced by many who make an adequate immune response to the agent and have no sequelae from the encounter. Their immunological knowhow, in the form of antibodies, may lead to the clearance of the same ubiquitous but unknown virus that has not been handled well by the immune system of CFS sufferers. We have no evidence to support this theory, but the reaction in muscles that can follow an infusion of gammaglobulin evoke images of antibodies getting into muscles and attacking something.

Alternatively, gammaglobulin may correct a defect in the immuno-regulatory T cells that then return to the business of getting their house in order. Part of this involves the eradication of viruses or virus particles in brain and nervous tissue.

Dealing with hundreds of patients with CFS brings one face to face with many of the inadequacies of modern medicine. For those of us who teach medicine it is saddening to realise that we have produced a generation of physicians, so delighted with what they know and so comfortable with high-technology investigation that they spend insufficient (if any) time in considering medical science's ignorance of so much of the body's ordered and disordered function.

Modern doctors regrettably prefer to look at the results on a piece of computer paper than to listen to the credible, consistent and reasoned observations of their patients who, after all, live with their bodies. If the blood tests are all normal, the symptoms are generated from a disturbed psyche.

This attitude on the part of doctors has led to exaggerated suffering, despair and even suicide among victims of CFS. The almost universal reaction of my patients with CFS when I show them their abnormal T cell results is to break into tears of relief. To be believed, to have some proof that they are not neurotic, results in an instant measure of improvement. 'Please, can I have a photocopy of the results?' is an almost universal request.

The other consequence of the intellectual arrogance of some of my colleagues has been the driving of patients with CFS and indeed all incurable and poorly understood diseases into the somewhat dangerous world of alternative medicine. Here, if one is lucky, one may find an innovative, intuitive and scientifically minded practitioner of a healing art that constructively challenges the orthodoxy of modern medicine. Unfortunately, however, one is far more likely to find oneself being treated by a scientifically unsound seller of hope to the hopeless, the easiest of targets for charlatans and the misguided. No group has been more exploited than patients with CFS who, in quite understandable and indeed predictable despair, will try anything.

Patients have flocked to New Zealand to a man who claims to cure CFS by exposing one to a specific sequence of colours. Others have been fed massive amounts of vitamin C, tryptophan, lecithin, macrobiotics, cod liver oil, etc. One American healer claims that CFS can be cured by tapping repeatedly over the thymus gland and summoning, with all one's mental energy, the T cells that lurk within. Patients can spend $3000 or so to go to detoxification units to be purified by enemas, vitamins and exercise. One poor patient of mine recently spent a lot of money purchasing variously shaped crystals that she placed strategically around her bed as instructed so as to draw upon the ancient and mystical powers of the Egyptian pyramids which can exorcise the evils that produce CFS.

The therapy and therapists survive only because of the fact that many patients in their desperation experience short-term improvement as the well known placebo effect influences those anxious to find a cure. Many who are helped are indeed psychologically disturbed patients for whom such way-out remedies are psychotherapy. Many of these patients feel and indeed reported that they had CFS, but in reality this is not the case.

Because of the nature of the symptoms many patients I see who are sure they have CFS are wrong. As we said previously the art of a physician as much as his science is needed to distinguish the organic from the functional and to realise that, while the treatment will differ, the suffering with both types of disorders will be the same.

Let me finish with an attempt to settle some of the controversial points about which we now feel certain. It is true that CFS can run in families but almost certainly for genetic, not infectious, reasons. Genetic programing of family members makes them susceptible to whatever is the disease-producing mechanism.

It is true that CFS rarely starts in patients over the age of fifty but definite cases do occur. It can affect middle-aged individuals and can persist well into their old age. It is certainly not true that CFS spares children; I have treated numerous children, the youngest being six years of age. It could well affect even younger children.

CFS is often reported in the media as a 'yuppie disease'. This is not only cruel but inaccurate. The connotation conjured up by the term is that of a successful young executive or professional who finds it all a bit too much and who needs an excuse to withdraw from the rat race. CFS affects peoples from all socioeconomic groups, though the persistence and contacts needed to clear a path through the prejudice and ignorance of many physicians may be more readily available to better-educated people.

It is true that CFS seems to affect many more women than men, as is true with most immunological diseases. When a man does suffer from CFS he usually has a very severe form of the illness.

A number of patients with symptoms consistent with CFS claim to be extremely sensitive to the environment and the numerous chemicals found in food, drugs, etc. Is such chemical sensitivity (that, whatever its cause, is definitely not allergic in the immunological sense) an extension of the basic CFS syndrome? Do similar mechanisms to those that affect muscle and nervous tissue interfere with biochemical events that detoxify incoming chemicals? I do not know the answers to these questions but have a completely open mind on the matter. Most people with CFS do not have extreme sensitivity to chemicals but those who do are even more incapacitated than patients for whom fatigue and changes in mental function predominate. Much more research is needed before we can say if this is a separate disease or part of the CFS spectrum.

To summarise, many people throughout the world, perhaps indeed 1 per cent to 1.5 per cent of all people suffer from a syndrome the constant feature of which is an extraordinary, almost indescribable muscle fatigue that makes even the most minimal exercize difficult. This syndrome also features neurological disturbances, most commonly resulting in headaches, confusion, defects in concentration, short-term memory and emotional lability.

This problem can sweep through a community in an epidemic form when it is most likely that an as-yet-undiscovered virus is responsible and many, though certainly not all individuals meeting the virus, will be affected. A less severe form of the virus may produce endemic disease that may select individuals who are genetically predisposed because of a weakness in the immune system's ability to handle this particular virus. Alternatively, this syndrome may be triggered by stimulating a disordered immune system. If this is the case, many non-infectious agents and micro-organisms other than viruses may be responsible. Viruses or virus particles may change the function of cells in muscles and the nervous system either directly or indirectly.

Recent evidence has established the organic nature of the problem. It is associated with a disordered immune system and the possibility that many, perhaps most, patients can be helped by immunotherapy is exciting. That the mysterious mechanisms responsible for this disease will be revealed to medical science in the near future is a more-than-reasonable prediction.

In the meantime, it is essential that we spread this new knowledge throughout the medical and lay community alike so that thousands of sufferers of CFS can be given the appropriate sympathy and encouragement and indeed hope that may make their suffering bearable as we move ever closer to the definitive cure for this disabling disease.

PART V ASSISTING THE WARRIORS

10 | Some weapons of the immunologist

AROUND the visitors' quarters at the university where I was working in Dakar, Senegal, was one of the poorest 'suburbs' of a poor city. Seven hundred and fifty thousand people lived in tin shanties and mud huts. In this area there is no sewerage and no running water for individual shacks. There are at frequent intervals, in corners of intersecting unpaved streets, water pumps from which the precious fluid is collected and carried home in all kinds of vessels.

One afternoon I was strolling down such a street in the middle of which were playing perhaps twelve to fifteen boys of about ten years of age. They were enjoying their beloved soccer, running with endless enthusiasm after the tired soccer ball that bounced at crazy angles from the ruts in the road. No fear of being run over here; goats on the road were more of a menace than automobiles. A noisy, happy and very dusty scene.

As I approached the boys, one of them, a ten-year-old called Ibrahima, kicked a soccer ball to his friends and ran to a corner water pump. With one hand he pumped some water into his other hand and sipped the none-too-sterile liquid, splashing some on his hot and dusty face. As he was leaning down to enjoy his refreshment, a dog appeared from nowhere and, quite unprovoked, rushed at the little boy and nipped the back of his neck. As a result of the bite the skin on the back of Ibrahima's neck was broken and oozed blood immediately.

Naturally, the bitten child screamed. His soccer mates, many of whom had witnessed the attack, fell into a shocked silence for a few seconds and then started yelling loudly as they ran off in different directions; clearly, they wished to distance themselves from that dog as quickly as possible. Ibrahima stood frozen to the spot and bolted up the street, right into the arms of his father who had come outside together with a number of other adults to investigate the cause of the commotion.

Much shouting from the adults ensued and the father disappeared into his shack, to emerge seconds later with a towel in one hand and a large knife in the other. With the towel wrapped around his left hand and forearm he approached the dog responsible for the attack.

Now the dog in question was of course a stray, one of thousands of emaciated, indeed pathetic-looking animals that wander the dusty streets in these parts. Dirty brown fur covered much of his body but a number of areas, particularly on his back, were bare and indeed ulcerated. The dog was a distressing sight. After its 'attack' it had not moved. It stood, head down, looking slowly from left to right as if it could not make up its mind whether to catch some of the water drops still falling from the pump.

Urged on by the instant crowd, now surging all around me, the father slowly approached the hapless animal. I remember thinking that the father's revengeful intentions were somewhat extreme. I knew little of Africans then or I would have realised how out of character such a motive would have been. That the father was desperate to save his son's life never entered my head.

The dog made no attempt to move as the father fell upon it; the animal appeared to be in a trance, in fact. The big black arm partially covered by the towel encircled the neck of the surprisingly placid dog and in a second the large knife had cut the animal's throat. Blood spurted into the dusty street ahead of the animal as the father carefully positioned himself with legs astride the dog's back. The animal died instantly but before my horrified and perplexed eyes the father continued to saw away at the dog's throat. In seconds his large knife had decapitated the animal. The head was quickly wrapped in the towel that had previously protected the father's arm and the dog's carcass was left in the gutter to be instantly attended to by a million ever-ready flies.

Throughout this drama the street resounded to yells of fear, advice and congratulations. Someone, perhaps Ibrahima's mother, was washing his neck with what looked like a bar of soap. It was at this point that I was noticed. The father, who of course did not know me let alone know I was a doctor, hurried up to me and explained. *'Monsieur, monsieur! Je pense que le chien rage! Avez-vous une voiture? Il me faut porter la tête à l'hôpital'.*

Suddenly the scene made sense. The father was convinced that the dog had rabies, a very common problem in this part of the world. The local population had been taught that animals that bite must be killed and their head transported *'immediatement'* to the hospital for an examination of the animal's brain. Anxious to help, and fascinated, I took the father and a few supporters to the hospital with the dog's head wrapped in the now very messy towel. Ibrahima, strangely enough, was left behind with his mother.

At the hospital the head was checked in with details about the incident. Father was instructed to return for the results of the pathology test two days later. Muttering that he knew the results would confirm the fact that the wretched dog had rabies, he headed for home while I had myself educated at the hospital.

Rabies is one of the most lethal of infections, but there are measures that can be taken to help people who are at risk of developing this infection after a bite. The problem is that the treatment is somewhat risky, hence the need to be sure of the diagnosis before commencing someone on preventative therapy.

A million Americans are bitten by animals every year; this is a common problem throughout the world. After every bite from an animal one must consider whether anti-rabies therapy is warranted. Skunks, wolves, raccoons, mongooses and bats can all be responsible for spreading this disease. In the poorer parts of the world, however, wild dogs are mainly responsible.

Rabies is caused by a tiny virus excreted in the saliva of infected animals. Once it finds itself under the skin of, for example, someone who has been bitten, it burrows into the nerves in the skin and then literally marches along those nerves up the spinal cord into the brain where it can cause terrible damage. It may take twelve days or twelve months to reach the brain, hence the clinical picture following infection varies considerably.

Rabies is lethal; only three humans are known to have survived an established brain infection. The paralysis of muscles needed for swallowing that is a feature of the infection, means that saliva will accumulate in the mouth and eventually spill out; hence 'frothing at the mouth'. While only five people a year die of rabies in the USA, probably fifteen thousand or more die of this infection worldwide.

In countries where rabies is a problem, all domestic dogs should be vaccinated against the virus as this very much reduces the risks of humans getting the disease. Dogs are more likely than humans to wander unprotected into the woods and be bitten by wild animals. Thousands of proud owners have their dogs vaccinated against rabies every year and indeed, have them similarly protected against other scourges such as distemper (dog measles), yet few of those owners would ever stop to think about the extraordinary benefits vaccines have brought to humankind and animalkind.

Why don't we make vaccines to all the infectious diseases that plague humans? Because getting the agents into a suitable form for introduction to the immune system is not easy. Many viruses are hard to grow in the laboratory in sufficient amounts to produce commercial quantities of vaccine. Indeed, many viruses have defied all our attempts to kill them and yet have them remain good stimulants of the immune system.

Take rabies, for example. This is a difficult virus to culture; until recently it could be grown only in duck embryos. The virus grown in bulk in this fashion is then inactivated chemically. This is a delicate reaction, however, and there is still a slight risk of developing severe neurological disease after vaccination. This complication rate used to occur as frequently as one in every six thousand vaccinations. It is now in the order of one in one hundred thousand with the duck embryo vaccine. An even newer vaccine, made by growing the virus in abnormal human cells, is apparently even less risky and seems set to replace the duck embryo vaccine. However, pain at the injection site, fever and nausea continue to be problems associated with the vaccine. For adequate protection, multiple injections are needed. The duck embryo vaccine, the only one available in Africa, does not give one hundred per cent protection, while the newer vaccine appears to be more efficient as no failures have been reported to date.

Back to poor Ibrahima, nursing a sore neck and hating dogs as he awaited the results of the tests on his attacker's brain.

At the hospital the pathologist called a colleague at the Institut Pasteur, a French research and vaccine-producing institute based in Paris but with branches in many Third World countries. The Institute had the equipment needed for the test.

A piece of the dog's brain was removed and rapidly frozen. While in this state a wafer-thin slice was cut with an extremely sharp blade and the frozen piece of tissue laid on a glass slide. The slide was then coated with a preparation known to contain antibody against the rabies virus. If rabies was there the antibody would find it. The antibody was tagged with a dye that emits a bright green color when stimulated with ultra-violet light. Green spots in the brain mean virus. The dog's tissue was brilliantly green, so loaded with virus had it become.

Ibrahima was brought to the hospital and examined. He had a fever and a sore neck but seemed otherwise okay. Into the area of the wound he was given an injection of serum containing antibodies to the virus. The Centre for Disease Control in the United States has been collecting blood from volunteers who have been immunised against rabies. This blood, would, of course, contain high levels of antibody against the virus. Their serum was packaged as hyper-immune antirabies gamma-globulin and shipped around the world. It was, however, in short supply and was therefore precious. It was not to be used unless the diagnosis was clear.

This preparation gives a form of instantaneous protection, a gift from one human to another. In addition to the antibodies, Ibrahima was given an injection of the rabies vaccine. A large amount of killed virus would rapidly stimulate his T and B cells to make a vigorous response to the agent that had almost certainly been injected by the rabid dog.

The ending to this story is a happy one as Ibrahima did not develop rabies and may one day grow to be a great soccer star, thanks to modern immunology.

Passive protection

We must explore a little further the concept of passive protection, in contradistinction to the active protection induced by immunisation.

In 1668, Sir Christopher Wren, very busy rebuilding London after its great fire, was asked to design a needle that could be used in experiments aimed at determining the feasibility or otherwise of transferring blood from one animal to another. He promptly designed the hypodermic needle which is still in use today.

Samuel Pepys records in his diaries that a successful demonstration of the needle took place at the home of a doctor in London. Blood was indeed passed from one animal to another. (Presumably the transfused animal did not die, for it is not mentioned, but if it did not, it was very lucky as the blood it received would almost certainly have been incompatible.) One of the doctors at the demonstration, so Pepys tells us, said to the assembled throng, 'I feel this is the beginning of a new era that will see the mending of bad blood by the borrowing from a better body.'

So was born into medicine the concept of passive protection, long used by Nature. Maternal antibody crosses the placenta to fill up babies with antibodies made against troublesome germs that the mother has seen during the months of her pregnancy. This is a gift to tide babies over until they can make their own antibodies. From the last decade of the nineteenth century, passive protection in this form has been used in medicine.

At first serum from horses was used. Old horses were immunised with substances that were dangerous to humans such as diphtheria and then, after they had had time to make a lot of antibody, serum was collected from the animals. This was then administered to patients at risk of developing the infection. Diphtheria, at the time, was one of the most serious killers. Patients were definitely protected in this way but as you can imagine, giving horse serum to humans provokes its own set of problems. Our immune systems react to the 'foreignness' that we recognise in these equine proteins.

Today we use human serum collected from subjects who have either recovered from or have been immunised against a particular infectious agent. Immune serum of this nature is available to help protect us from tetanus, hepatitis B, rabies, mumps, pertussis or whooping cough and chicken pox. You may be surprised to know that we still use some serum containing potent antibodies obtained from immunised animals. Animals supply us with antibodies against diphtheria, those organisms that cause fatal food poisoning or botulism, the venom of the black widow spider and certain snake and scorpion poisons.

Another form of passive protection is needed by the many patients who cannot make antibodies at all; that is, patients with antibody deficiency disease. Blood is pooled from 3000 to 20,000 healthy donors and the serum extracted. It is then concentrated in a form that contains almost pure IgG. This can be given intravenously to patients who need it. Monthly infusions for life of this gift 'from a better body' allow such patients to lead an almost normal life.

Active protection

In the United States of America most children receive the full benefits of the best vaccines because there are laws that stop children from going to school unless they are adequately protected and hence will not act as a source of infection for others. In many Western countries, where these vaccines can be afforded, sad to say immunisation is not compulsory. Those countries continue to have children and therefore adults who suffer from horrible complications of common infectious diseases.

All babies should begin their assisted defense of self at two months of age with an injection of a vaccine mixture containing diphtheria, pertussis and tetanus antigens (DPT shot). In addition, they should swallow a little polio vaccine. Babies should then receive booster doses of the same antigens at four and six months. At that point the child is fully protected against these four diseases.

At fifteen months of age children should be given another combination of antigens. This one contains measles, mumps and rubella (German measles) viruses. They will be protected for life from these diseases following successful vaccination. At eighteen months of age, I recommend a further booster dose of DPT and polio and then a final one at seven years of age. Tetanus shots should be given every ten years throughout life.

Diphtheria is caused by infection with *corynebacterium diphtheriae*. The bacteria penetrate the back of the throat and there may produce a powerful toxin that can paralyse nerves. From the throat this poison may spread rapidly around the body. The bacteria, interestingly enough, do this because they are infected with a virus that makes them do it. So, with diphtheria you get two infections at once. People of all ages who are not protected die of diphtheria; about thirty people a year in the USA. Generally, they come from isolated communities where they have escaped the attention of immunologists.

Tetanus, in which a painful spasm and then paralysis of muscles causes death, is produced by the release of a neuro toxin from *clostridium tetani*; an ubiquitous organism found in the soil everywhere and commonly in animal excreta. The organism lies dormant in the ground in the form of spores that become activated when they enter a wound. In many Third World countries there is still an unfortunate habit of placing cow dung around the stump of a baby's severed umbilical cord. Many infants die of tetanus as a result. As many as three hundred cases of tetanus can occur in the United States in any one year and seventy per cent of these patients will die. No region of the USA is spared.

Whooping cough can, and does, kill infants. Until recently 10,000 cases were recorded annually in the USA. With adequate immunisation no child should die of this disease. Severe complications and death usually follow infection of the brain and lungs. As whooping cough takes a severe toll on the very young, immunisation must start as soon as feasible. Recent epidemics among adults in England and Australia clearly demonstrate that when immunisation is not compulsory, the infectious agent will survive in the community and infect adults immunised as a child, but whose immunity is now waning. For this reason, adults in such countries are well advised to have a small booster dose of this vaccine. On the other hand, in countries where the whole community is immunised against pertussis, so little of the infectious agent survives in the community that even the odd person who has escaped vaccination is protected.

Today paralytic polio is rare in countries where vaccine is freely available. In underdeveloped countries it remains a terrible curse. To see how effective this vaccine is you need only to remember that 15,000 cases of paralytic polio occurred annually in the USA during the 1950s. Today fewer than thirty cases are reported each year. It is a tragedy and a shameful reflection on the Western world's desertion of their brothers in the Third World that thousands of children will yet be crippled by this virus. Underdeveloped countries simply cannot afford to buy the vaccine.

In the USA in 1962, there were at least 500,000 cases of measles. In 1972 the number was less than 40,000 cases. In 1974, measles vaccination slackened off; fewer than 60 per cent of children were immunised, and as a result a major epidemic broke out in 1977. Measles can be fatal. Five to fifteen per cent of victims develop secondary bacterial infections and one in a thousand cases develop a potentially fatal infection of the brain. Measles should not be taken lightly. In underdeveloped countries it remains a major killer of children under the age of three.

Mumps is caused by a virus that replicates in glandular tissues. While it is usually mild, complications are frequent enough to make vaccination advisable. Mumps is a serious risk for boys who have reached puberty.

Twenty per cent develop a viral infection in their testicles than can sterilise them. Such infections are painful and incapacitating complications. Mumps is a leading cause of meningitis and brain inflammation and is also suspected to be one of the viruses that can cause diabetes.

Rubella or German measles is a mild disease of children and young adults. It would not warrant much attention except that rubella during pregnancy is associated with an extremely high risk of having an abnormal baby. Only by having everybody immunised can the amount of virus circulating in a community be contained and the tragedy of the congenital rubella syndrome be eradicated. A vaccine was developed in the USA after thousands of blind, deaf and mentally retarded and/or immunodeficient children were born in 1964 as a result of congenital rubella infection. The virus in the vaccine itself, although not dangerous to children or adults, is dangerous to the fetus and therefore cannot be given to pregnant women.

In answer to the question 'Lord, what must I do to have the perfect immune system?', the answer must be, 'First, pick thy parent very carefully.' Not the most practical of advice, maybe, but there is a message here nonetheless. You want both parents to come from at least three generations of octogenarians. No allergies, or immune diseases (especially diabetes and rheumatoid arthritis) and no cancer in the family, please. If you have such parents, husband your assets carefully, as you are destined for senior citizenship.

If you do not have such parents, do not despair; much can be done and your fundamental genetic flaws may be fixable. We live in an age where genetic engineering, already so useful for examining the basic defects in disease and having bacteria make endless supplies of insulin and the like, will soon be used for therapy. Genetic information can be spliced into chromosomes, adding a new program to the genetic repertoire already present, or correcting one that is defective. If we can splice into a bacterial chromosome the blueprints for making human insulin, we will soon be able to splice into the bone marrow cells of children making an abnormal hemoglobin the genes that will tell that child's cells how to make normal hemoglobin. If there is a second edition to this book, genetic engineering will undoubtedly need to be given the fullest coverage. For now, however, we will turn our attention to other immediately available strategies.

What is the best way of extending the healthy lifespan of caged rats? The answer is to deprive them of some of the calories they wish to consume, that is, mild starvation. Rats can experience thirty to sixty per cent increase in their lifespan if you restrict the intake of calories from birth. The same is true for mice who, on such a regimen, look like four-month-old mice when they are actually sixteen months old. As mice only live for two years, you can see the significance of this observation.

In addition to living longer, the animals in the above experiments were found to be more resistant to infection and cancer. Thymic involution, that inbuilt curtain on the immune drama, is markedly delayed in the underfed. Why should this be?

While admitting that we do not have all the answers to this riddle, some interesting facts have emerged. Rats do not overeat in the way humans do and obese rats are as rare as obese snakes. (There are strains of chickens that become obese; interestingly enough, they have an immunological disease of their thyroid glands.) Animals eat appropriately. Restricting the calories available to rats keeps them lean, of course, but it also decreases some of the immunoregulatory activity of T cells. These rats can therefore make a more vigorous response to infection, etc. What harmful effects may be associated with this 'therapy' is not certain as we cannot gauge rat wellbeing very well; certainly no gross abnormalities occur.

While most nutritionists feel that Western man, at least, eats a poorly balanced diet containing far too much fat, you only have to look around you to see that apart from eating a poorly balanced diet, we simply eat too much; obese humans are not hard to find. Studies of the immune system of the obese have, in fact, been done. The ability of their neutrophils to swallow and kill bacteria is reduced. The killing power of their T cells is damaged. Frequently they are deficient in zinc and magnesium, two elements essential for normal immune performance. The obese suffer from more infections that tend to be more serious.

Would we live longer, healthier lives if we were minimally starved like the rats? Probably, but controlled experiments with humans to settle this issue are hard to organise, as you can imagine.

On the other hand, humankind's inhumanity ensures that we have abundant clinical material with which to determine the effects of real starvation on the immune response. It is dramatic. In Third World countries malnutrition, especially the loss of calories from good protein sources, rapidly takes immune performance through any stage of heightened adequacy and plunges it into despair.

Antibody capacity is lost first and, with that, defenses against bacteria crumble. Gastroenteritis becomes a way of life, pus oozes from infected eyes and skin. T cells remain a little longer, then they also fail. All the magical defense mastery we had discussed at length vanishes. To compound the tragedy, food, when and it if arrives, does not correct the defects instantly; far from it. It may take months or even years to return T cell function to normal.

Deprived of food and hence immunological help, the parasites that infest the Third World take over and the human suffering that results is indescribable.

In our time, television cameras depict the horrors of the end stages of starvation well but not perfectly. You can see the suffering and you can hear the exhausted sobs of the starved, but you cannot smell it or feel it. The smell is very definitely one of death: death achieved and death approaching.

The feeling is one of utter despair, no faint glimmer of hope is seen in the eyes of adults and children. No longer do exhausted hands brush the flies away. No longer do failing minds pay any attention to another group of healthy-looking doctors moving in their midst with no real help in their hands.

I had the distressing experience of visiting starving tribes in Africa with medicine and vaccines to dispense, but no food; a useless exercise in frustration. What is so clear to those who get a chance to work in such areas is that the world cannot afford to have millions of people chronically malnourished and disease-ridden. Leaving human sympathy aside for the moment, the loss of productivity, the resultant destruction of potentially arable soil and the spread of disease will cost all of us dearly. It is very much in our own interest to end the cycle of poverty and disease that affect so many of our brothers and sisters.

Specific vitamin deficiencies significantly compromise immune performance. Patients with Vitamin A deficiency find it hard to make IgA. The binding power of their antibodies is reduced. Lower numbers of circulating lymphocytes are frequently found. With Vitamin C deficiency, protein synthesis is impaired and all the cells of the immune system perform less adequately. In addition, wound healing is significantly reduced. People suffering from a lack of sufficient vitamin B in their diet cannot make good delayed hypersensitivity reactions. They cannot reject grafted tissue normally. This deficiency, of course, is a very common problem among the alcoholics in our society.

Other deficiencies that significantly depress our immunological defenses result from a lack of iron, folic acid, zinc, riboflavin, niacin and magnesium. The last three are very important if we are to make antibody normally. Let me hasten to stress, however, that there is no evidence that the taking of very large amounts of any of these nutritionally essential materials improves immunological performance.

If some part of your unhappy anatomy is red, hot, swollen and painful, that part is said to be inflamed. The process producing the changes is called inflammation. Inflammation affects tissues, joints and, indeed, any part of the body and results from the release of chemicals that open up blood vessels in a particular area. The aim of the process is to allow antibodies and cells to move into an infected site. If that is the price we have to pay to overcome a potentially serious infection, well, so be it. But if that inflammation should turn out to be useless, indeed harmful, as it would in an autoimmune disease, we physicians must try and suppress it. The most powerful antiinflammatory drugs we possess are called steroids and of these the most potent are corticosteroids; perhaps you know them as hydrocortisone or prednisone.

Corticosteroids are produced in the cortex (outer areas, hence *cortico* steroids) of the tiny adrenal glands that sit astride the top of your kidneys. These chemicals are indispensable; without them we die. They are one of the body's prime catalysts, activating many processes from protein synthesis to the coloration of skin. In essence steroids drive forward a cell's intentions and thus may promote some happenings in the body and *suppress* others. Each morning our brain secretes a chemical that tells the adrenal gland to pour out adequate amounts of these precious hormones.

As you probably know, giving large amounts of hydrocortisone to patients can produce a miraculous melting away of disease processes caused by inflammation. Unfortunately, large doses given for a long time produce many side effects. Steroids interact with too many of the body's processes, so the results of their administration are many in number. Steroids used with knowledge and therefore appropriately are wonderful tools for reducing suffering. They can control asthma, help in the cure of leukemia and, most importantly, block inflammation.

Some doctors are irresponsible in their use of these potent drugs. In Italy many doctors give them to patients who are suffering from nothing more serious than the flu. This is a bad idea as steroids can, in fact, minimise the body's fight against the virus. On the other hand, there are doctors who refuse to use them at all, feeling that the side effects are too troublesome. Both approaches are erroneous. If the disease is more dangerous and distressing than the side effects of the drugs, the tradeoff is reasonable. In reality, many patients can have their lives made bearable, indeed enjoyable, on doses of corticosteroids that produce only minimal side effects.

Steroids in small doses block two actions of other chemicals released from neutrophils (the phagocytic and infection-swallowing cells) and the mast cells and basophils that release histamine and other blood vessel-dilating substances. In very large doses they can be immunosuppressive in the sense that they damage or even kill lymphocytes.

The major side effects may be stunting of growth, weight gain, especially in the cheeks, upper arms and top of the back, weakening of bones as calcium is displaced, easy bruising, changeable moods, increased appetite, ulcers, cataracts in the eyes, a higher than normal blood pressure and increased hair growth on the skin. In addition, the adrenal glands become very sluggish when one takes these drugs, for they need not produce hormones themselves. Consequently, stopping the drug after a long period of therapy can be dangerous; slow withdrawal is mandatory.

While steroids in high doses can affect lymphocytes, the antigen-recognising cells of the immune system, we seldom use them for this purpose. When it is necessary to suppress lymphocyte function (never a happy occurrence) we do have drugs that are capable of doing just that. Of the three most commonly used drugs, two, cyclophosphamide and azathioprine, are borrowed from cancer doctors who use them to block tumor growth. The third and most interesting, cyclosporine A, is a drug with unique properties.

Before we discuss these drugs let us look at situations where it would be necessary to cripple lymphocyte performance. The easiest situation to come to grips with involves organ transplantation.

A man who is now dependent on someone else's heart cannot be allowed to reject it. He must be immunosuppressed, despite the risks associated with non-specific depression of lymphocyte performance. If he cannot reject the heart that he has been given, he will not be able to reject normally those infections that might afflict him. We immunologists long for the day when we can 'tolerise' such a patient, that is, teach him to accept as 'self' those foreign antigens associated with his new heart while instructing him to continue to reject anything else foreign that comes his way.

Transplantation of vital organs is as dramatic a scenario as modern medicine can present, but it is a minor part of medicine, as very few patients are helped in this manner. Much more common are the autoimmune diseases we have discussed already. Take rheumatoid arthritis, for example. At least four per cent of the entire population suffer from this disease and occasionally in the worst examples we must suppress a patient's immune system.

Raymond was wheeled into my clinic in a wheelchair. A man of thirty-four, married with one child, and a retired schoolteacher, he was thin and miserable from long days of pain and frustration. Five years earlier, while supplementing his income, Ray had a job in a timber yard on weekends. At twenty-nine, healthy, happy and hardworking, he appeared to have a happy future.

One morning he picked up a pair of large wire cutters to remove a metal band wrapped very tightly around a bundle of timber. As he cut the tense band it gave way suddenly and fiercely, with the result that his wrist was cruelly twisted. A painful tear of the tendons around the joint occurred. Two weeks later, not only had his hand not recovered, but other joints in his body had become swollen, hot and painful. Ray had developed rheumatoid arthritis, a disease wherein the joints are attacked and destroyed by misguided lymphocytes failing to recognise the joints as a part of self. In genetically disposed individuals, it is not unusual to have such events triggered by a traumatic episode such as the one described.

Five years later Ray was a cripple, weak, thin, anemic, chronically fatigued and for much of his time, wheelchair bound. He had been treated aggressively by experienced people. Aspirin, gold, steroid injections into his joints, penicillamine, and every new antiinflammatory drug that was marketed had been tried, with little effect. Now we discussed the risks of suppressing his immune response with cyclophosphamide, a potent but dangerous drug that many of us who deal with the severest form of this disease find useful. I explained to Ray that his T and B cells were actively damaging his joints. It was clear that some permanent damage had already occurred but even more damage would occur if the disease was not controlled.

Cyclophosphamide is a drug that kills cells when they try and divide to produce more of themselves. Cell division is an essential component of an immunological attack. The cells that divide most rapidly are the ones most affected. In immune systems the cells that divide most rapidly are antibody-producing cells or B cells; they are inhibited by these drugs.

We went on to discuss the benefits of blocking the attack on his joints with the drugs and, of course, the side effects that he might encounter. The most serious side effect is sterility; it was very unlikely that Ray would ever be able to father another child after taking the drug for a few weeks. The rapidly dividing sperm-producing cells in the testes are killed.

I could see that this was a blow for he only had the one child and the family longed for a second. Today we would store his semen for future use by artificial insemination. At the time, however, we were not doing this. After much discussion and time for consideration of all that was involved, Ray decided to take the drug. The disease was worse than any potential side effects.

Not all patients with rheumatoid arthritis respond to this drug, but Ray did. His disease seemed to largely disappear in his first months on therapy. He left his wheelchair and cried at the joy of being able to walk freely. Not that he was perfect. Some structural damage could not be reversed. Ray lost his hair for a few months, he was sterilised by the treatment as predicted but he was able to return to his profession. The psychological benefits of being gainfully employed again might even have exceeded his happiness at having his arthritis subside. He continues to do well although he will always need the most meticulous medical attention if he is to securely walk the tightrope that is suspended between a flareup of his disease and a dangerous degree of immunosuppression.

Of all the immunosuppressive drugs the most exciting is the newest to be developed; cyclosporine A. This drug is produced by a fungus and is a tiny chemical that packs a huge punch. It has the so far unique ability to stop T cells from secreting interleukin 2 (IL2). You may remember that IL2 is the pivotal chemical that gives permission for all other cells in the immune system to attack. This drug has revolutionised the transplant business as it makes non-rejection of donated organs almost certain. The drug brings us closer to the idea of having chemicals that will affect only the cells we wish to target, other tissues being unaffected. Cyclosporine does affect the liver and the kidneys and can only be used for three months without concern for side effects, leading many of us to switch to other agents. Intense research is being carried out to produce a drug with similar effect on the immune system which will not be toxic to other cells even with prolonged use.

Immunologists can use naturally occurring and potent chemicals that drive forward or alter immunological responses. We now have on our therapeutic shelves interleukin 2 (some of which is produced by friendly bacteria after some genetic trick), interferon, thymic hormones and a myriad of small chemicals extracted from healthy T cells. These factors are not specific for any one person and therefore are of great value in modifying immunological responses. We use these for patients with immunodeficiency, chronic viral infections and cancer.

Clinical immunologists are experimenting with a number of potentially exciting ways of helping patients with immunological diseases. Watch the developments with the technique known as total lymphoid irradiation. Here, by giving gamma irradiation to all lymph nodes in the body, we seem to be able to return the immune system to a fetal-like state in which it may be possible to re-establish tolerance to self that has been lost and is resulting in serious disease. Antigens that were being treated as foreign may again be respected as self. This treatment is proving particularly valuable in its early experimental phases for patients with multiple sclerosis, rheumatoid arthritis and systemic lupus erythematosis.

Watch also for progress in the food allergy business. At last we are purifying the antigens from food that actually cause the allergic response. Once these are purified, our ability to diagnose and treat the misery produced by food allergy will be very much improved.

As is true with all significant areas of human advancement, science needs its theoreticians as well as its development specialists, that is, people who can take an hypothesis, prove it and utilise the result. Immunology is no exception. One of the great theoreticians of our time was the Australian Nobel Laureate Macfarlane Burnett who influenced me and hundreds of other young would-be scientists as we learned our craft. When I knew him he had officially retired but was nonetheless only too happy to discuss experimental results with those of us around him. Interpretation of observed data was for him a great game of chess. How many ways could you make that result mean something? How many new experiments could you demand as a result of your life's efforts?

Burnett was a great theoretician who understood autoimmunity before anyone else. He realized that scientific truths would have to be established in slow, often painful A to B to C fashion but this was not his way. A to L and then on to S was his way; let someone else come along and prove that your ideas were correct and fill in the missing pieces of the puzzle. They would have an honorable second prize. 'Don't cross Ts and dot Is,' he told me time and time again.

I first met his good friend and intellectual adversary Niels Jerne at a scientific birthday party to honor Burnett's seventieth year. These men were, and Jerne continues to be at this writing, the giants of theoretical immunology. Nothing pleased either man more than to come up with a theory that challenged contemporary beliefs and then have someone else prove that they were 100 per cent correct.

It was in this spirit that Jerne produced his 'network' theory. In essence what he proposed was this. When we make an antibody to, for example, a part of the tetanus toxoid that might be injected into us after an injury, the antibody does all the things you would now expect of it. But, said Jerne, those antibodies become antigens. Their presence will make our bodies make antibodies to them, that is, anti-antibodies!

Surely this time Jerne had gone too far; our antibodies are self and should not promote a response from any of our cells. Strange or not, claimed Jerne, you will find that we make antibodies to antibodies and that such antibodies will provoke a third antibody, etc.

Imagine you are in a small boat in the middle of a lake and you heave a big stone into the middle of all that confined water. Shock waves will race to the shore and back again causing visible ripples to appear on the surface as the waves collide. Little by little the ripples get smaller until they fade away completely. That is what happens when you throw an antigen into the body, claimed Jerne; waves of antibodies are formed against each other, each new one provoking a little less of a response than the one before so that the process gradually dampens down and disappears.

I would not be telling you this story if Jerne had not been correct. Fascinating to report, however, there is more to this phenomenon than just the rippling affect. Anti-antibodies interact with specific T cells that can regulate the production by B cells of the first antibody. Being able to harness this form of immunological reaction will provide us with exciting therapeutic possibilities. If you had available antibodies to specific antibodies, you could stop the body's production of those specific antibodies. We will look at some examples shortly.

In our ignorance at the moment we just have to accept the fact, now well established, that our immune system makes an exception to its 'no reactivity to self' rule when it comes to antibodies. More accurately, we

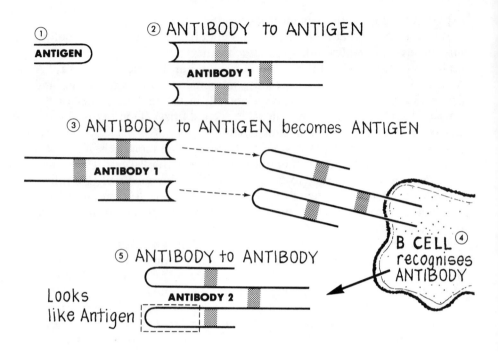

are reacting to just one part of the antibody when we produce anti-antibodies. That part of the antibody that is antigenic is called the idiotype. This is the portion of the molecule that has combined with the antigen, that is, the portion of the antibody with the three-dimensional configuration that is perfectly moulded to the shape of the antigen: the key (antigen) in the lock (antibody) analogy we have discussed earlier. Antibodies to this 'lock' are called anti-idiotypic antibodies.

Let's see how we can apply Jerne's discovery. Imagine you are in a clinical immunologist's office in a few years' time. Your problem is incapacitating ragweed allergy. Your immunologist explains to you, as he would today, that you have made an excessive amount of IgE antibody to ragweed. When the two combine on the surface of mast cells and basophils, histamine and other similar agents are released and you suffer hives, hay fever, asthma, etc.

In the future, he will add the following good news. We will have to turn off your production of IgE antibody against ragweed, or you will never get better. You are not making enough antibody to the IgE to keep its production moderate. We will give you some anti-idiotypic antibody, that is, antibody to that part of your IgE that recognizes ragweed and shut production down. This will be safe, specific and indeed sensational desensitisation.

One other use of anti-idiotypic antibodies is already with us. If you think of an antigen and an antibody using the lock and key analogy we discussed, we can take it one step further. If you make an antibody to the lock it will look like the key. In other words, the idiotypic region of the anti-idiotypic antibody will look like the antigen that started off the reaction in the first place. We can immunise animals and humans with anti-idiotypic antibodies and get the same response that we might get if we gave the antigen. The difference is that the antigens may be harmful. When we immunise people with live viruses (e.g., polio virus) there is always a chance that the attenuating process may not have been satisfactory and disease could develop. But administration of an antibody against antibodies to polio virus is harmless and yet effective.

These are but a few of the tools of the clinical immunologist currently in use or soon to be developed. It is an exciting area, for I do not exaggerate in saying that 80 per cent of all human suffering from disease could be wiped out by the mastery of the immune response.

11 | Reinforcements: the mind as an ally

MARTINA was fourteen and thin, better than being fourteen and fat she supposed, but her thinness worried both her and her mother. It is not that she was sick; far from it. She was a likely candidate for her school's track team. Her lack of padding was not due to poor eating habits either. She would outeat her sixteen-year-old brother every time. Everybody joked about her skinny frame and she hated it. She prayed that puberty would make a difference. At least if she developed some breast tissue, that would give her some shape.

Martina was not doing well at school despite working fairly hard and she had come to terms with her own (and everybody else's) conclusion that she was not too smart. Academic achievement or rather lack of it did not worry her, for her ambition, constant now for six months, was to travel the big wide world; the life of an airline stewardess was for her. Mother thought she was pretty enough and if she grew too tall for the jumbo jets she might just make it as a model. Skinny frames were great for hanging clothes on.

Martina, however, did have two big worries besides her lack of avoirdupois. Her brother David was taking drugs and no one else in the family knew. She had caught him sniffing some white powder into his nose. She was not stupid, and did not accept his claim that the stuff was medicine.

Her second worry was her mother. Although healthy-looking at the age of thirty-six, her mother had suffered from rheumatic fever as a child and the mitral valve in her heart had been damaged. Something about it was too narrow, she had heard many times, and her mother's heart had to pump very hard to push blood through a valve that had become a tiny hole. Twice her mother had undergone surgery to open the valve but each time, after a few years' improvement, it had closed down again.

Martina adored her mother and she could not bear to think of her pain if she knew how stupid David was being. She was about to have another operation; a new manmade valve would be sewn into her heart.

Then, quite unexpectedly, Martina's mother died on the operating table soon after her operation started. A blood clot or something had shot into her lungs and killed her. Martina's father told me later that his daughter screamed denial as he told her the news and then cried in pathetic despair for three never-ending days before total physical and emotional exhaustion led her into a restless sleep punctuated by body-shaking sobs.

Months later Martina told me how severe had been the shock, how painful the acute sense of loss. She felt cheated, not only because she had lost her best friend and mother, but also because she had had no reason to worry about the surgery and therefore no time to prepare herself for this loss. As a result those first weeks after Mother's death found her racked with despair, anger and guilt.

A sad story, of course, but had there been more to it than that I would not have subjected you to the details. No, the story and the suffering for this child were just beginning.

Two weeks to the day after her mother died, she woke to find her fingers and right shoulder painful and stiff. By noon the pain and stiffness were gone but by the same evening the pain had returned and was now in her right knee as well. Two days later she was a bedridden cripple. Excruciatingly painful and hot knees, ankles, shoulders and hands robbed her of her mobility.

Doctors examined the child. Tests were done on her blood and some fluid that was aspirated from her knee by a long needle connected to a syringe. A diagnosis was made: Martina had rheumatoid arthritis. The progression from track team candidate to cripple had taken a mere three days.

Five days later as her joints were improving slightly thanks to continued bedrest and medicines Martina noted she was passing a lot of urine. Every hour she would pass large amounts and the thirst that this produced made her drink constantly. After three days of this her thin frame looked like a skeleton with grossly disproportioned joints.

More tests, more doctors and a new diagnosis. Not only did Martina have rheumatoid arthritis, she had also developed diabetes mellitus. Diabetes occurs when our pancreas fails to secrete enough insulin. Insulin is needed to get sugar (energy) into our cells. If the sugar cannot get into cells, it circulates in the blood and must be removed by the kidneys. This they do well, but they must remove a lot of water from the blood to accomplish this, and hence one passes a lot of sweet urine. It is sweet because of the sugar, of course.

Perhaps Martina's psychic torture, racing around her brain in the form of frenzied electrical impulses, upset some delicate control mechanisms that actually operate far away from the cerebrum in distant joints and abdominal glands.

As both rheumatoid arthritis and diabetes are autoimmune diseases, i.e., disease in which the body's immune system attacks self-tissue as if it were foreign tissue, could this immunological turning against self be related in some strange way to a psychic turning against self?

Most experienced doctors could tell you stories similar to Martina's. I could tell you many more myself. I could tell you, for example, of a concert pianist who nearly died of bowel inflammation three weeks after breaking and permanently damaging a finger. I could detail the struggle for breath caused by an acute spasm in the airways of a forty-two-year-old mother who miscarried after six months of pregnancy. This was the closest she had come to fulfilling a now desperate dream of having a child. But instead of more stories let us look at some basic scientific facts as we see if we can convince ourselves that mind rules body and, in particular, that mind and immune system talk to each other constantly.

Charles Darwin was perhaps the first scientist to clearly enunciate the hypothesis that the mind, our intelligence-gathering and decision-making computer, can instantly and at will summon up a body response.

Darwin was fascinated by fear. Most people have been frightened. I do not enjoy fear myself, but some people love it and indeed will pay money to sit in the dark for two hours to be frightened. Like it or not, however, most people know fear produces a bodily response or responses almost as quickly as the mind tells us that a situation is scary.

A dangerous situation is recognised by the higher centers of the brain. A car is coming around the corner too fast, the driver will not be able to stop at the pedestrian crossing, we are only halfway across—danger! Now, if our minds compute these dangerous facts and tell us that we are in danger and yet do not automatically solve the problem for us, we will be struck by the car. We may die knowing what happened to us and regretting for a millisecond that we did not jump out of the way.

Fortunately, however, as Darwin appreciated, survival has demanded that mechanisms be developed whereby the appreciation of danger produces fear and fear produces an instantaneous bodily reaction. Our muscles tense and we *do* leap, most often successfully, to safety. Fright prepares us for flight. This wonderful mechanism obviously demands that a message races from the brain to the muscles and other vital organs.

The novelists of course have been describing these biological responses forever. Increased mental alertness in someone being terrorised may be related to us as, 'Hunted and desperate, his senses were as acute as those of a cat ready to pounce'. Activation of the nerves of the autonomic (automatic) nervous system that control the tiny muscles at the base of our hair follicles and the muscles that open and close blood vessels may be described as, 'Too late he saw the snake prepare to strike. The hair stood up on the back of his neck while the color drained from his face'.

The result of those messages from a frightened mind that affect the nerves controlling sweat glands and bowel contractions may be described as, 'His stomach was knotted with fear and beads of sweat formed on his brow as the executioner's gun was raised', etc.

Fear is good; fear is essential for it does marshal, with incredible speed, body responses that may save our life. But how is it that fear can instantly drain the color from one's cheeks by making superficial blood vessels in the skin spasm and therefore empty themselves of color?

The mind sends messages from the cerebral cortex, the most developed part of the brain, to other parts in one of two ways. Electrical messages can pass along the billions of telegraph wires that connect one vital part of the brain to another. Alternatively, chemicals may deliver messages as one part of the brain releases a substance that will activate some other part of the brain, while not affecting yet another region. We know how rapidly a chemical signal can work: how long does it take for some voluptuous perfume to conjure up a specific memory or anticipation in your brain?

But all this is going on inside our heads and to jump out of the way of that rapidly approaching car we need action in our legs. For some time now we have know that these peripheral responses involve not only electrical messages racing along nerves but the rapid release of hormones.

Hormones are the chemical products of the endocrine system, a system comprised of strategically placed glands that produce and store incredibly potent chemicals (hormones) that are released, when appropriate, to make us do something different. When you eat, within seconds, the pancreas gland releases insulin into the bloodstream to handle the sugar you have consumed. When a young man's genes tell him it's time to grow hair on his chest, his testicles will make and release testosterone and hair will sprout, muscles will strengthen and many other alterations will occur.

Not so long ago it was found that most of the hormones released around the body are controlled by a specific set of regulatory hormones released by the pituitary gland. This gland lives at the base of the brain. Put your finger at the top of your nose and point into your skull; just under the finger (under the bone, of course) sits the pituitary gland.

At the appropriate point in a woman's menstrual cycle, the pituitary gland sends a chemical message to the ovary, instructing it to release into the Fallopian tubes some eggs ready for fertilisation. The pituitary then waits for an egg to be fertilised. If it is not, the gland sends another message to the ovary, instructing the uterus to close down and shed the soft, warm and cosy lining built up in the uterus to nourish a young embryo. The woman then has a period: 'the weeping of a disappointed uterus'.

What has that to do with Martina's swollen joints? Patience, please, for just a little longer.

Recently it has been found that the pituitary gland itself is under the control of other hormones that come from a specific part of the brain called the hypothalmus which is intimately connected by chemical and electrical links to many of the brain's higher centers.

The glands that have received all the scientific publicity about 'fright, and flight' are the adrenals, on top of the kidneys. They produce two very important types of hormone: adrenalin, also called epinepherine, and steroids such as hydrocortisone. They are rightly called 'stress hormones' for their immediate release in times of danger is very important, but we now know that there are many others of equal importance.

Adrenalin makes the color drain from your face, not necessarily because Nature thinks there is an advantage in being pale. The advantage of having less blood flowing through the skin is that more blood flows into muscles, the muscles need blood for oxygen, oxygen gives them the energy needed to jump out of the way of the car, for example.

So far we have discussed fright leading to frantic messages being despatched around the body with physiological adjustments being made instantly so that we can respond appropriately. But novelists have often noted that this is not always the case . . .

'Marie saw him emerge from the shadows and recognised him instantly as the moon's light bathed his all too familiar face. She froze, terrified, mesmerised, her heart racing. She wanted to run, she wanted to scream but all she did was look into those cruel eyes as he approached her.'

What went wrong? Where was her hypothalmus when she needed it? Where were those electrical and chemical signals to her adrenal gland? We will never know and it is obviously likely that the monster had his way with her and then strangled the poor neuro-endocrine misfit.

'Too bad', said Darwin. 'Only the fittest survive and pass their genetic superiority to their offspring.'

Some of us confronted with situations of terror, respond appropriately, others do not.

Stress in any form; fear, bereavement, anger, etc., calls not only for hormonal alertness but also for immunological alertness. Suppose at the time we prepare for 'flight after fright' we engage the immunological system, another vital link in the defense of man. Some individuals may *enhance* their immune capacity when stressed, while others may damage its operations.

If that is so, then one could perhaps explain what happened to

Martina. Mental anguish led to inappropriate, indeed harmful, alterations in her hormonal and immune systems.

There is evidence that the central nervous system and immune system are linked, with hormones playing major roles as messengers connecting the higher centers of the brain to the immune system.

If you ask a biology student, 'Where do you find in the body the ability to "know thyself", the adaptability that allows for responses that are appropriate, not reflex, and memory capacity, which means that one can learn from experience and improve?' the answer in all likelihood will be 'The brain', with a quizzical look as to why one would ask such an easy question. In fact, the answer should be the brain and the immune system. The latter's ability to recognise self, adapt to circumstances and make specific responses as well as utilise memory capacity, bestows without doubt a certain intelligence on the immune system.

When something foreign enters the body, the immune response genes you inherited will determine whether you make an appropriate or inappropriate immune response. When one is stressed, coping response genes determine the stress response that you will make and whether that response is appropriate or inappropriate. Simply put, some people for genetic reasons handle, say, tuberculosis better than others; likewise, for genetic reasons, some handle tension better than others. We are exploring the possibility that the genetic knowledge for appropriateness in either situation is in some way linked. We would hypothesise that good coping genes are more likely to turn up in a patient who also has inherited good immune response genes.

We should back track for a minute and make sure that a couple of points already made are quite clear. Psychologists refer to an appropriate stress response as coping, in the way that an immunologist thinks of an immune response in terms of inflammation. We should also define how we are using the word 'stress' in our context. Stress is confusing as the noun can refer to the thing causing the stress (e.g., a situation) or to the response that situation provokes. Throughout, we use the term 'stress' to mean the situation that calls for a response from the person interpreting the situation.

Now scientists can study this subject in humans, and many do, but it is often easier to get at basic facts with animal observations and experiments. Let us look at the evidence, derived from animal studies, that suggests that the mind sends signals to the immune system and vice versa and that some of these signals arise from a perception of a stressful situation.

If you have read any behavioural physiology books you must have heard of the great Dr Pavlov and his equally famous dog. Pavlov knew of an unfortunate man who, at the end of the nineteenth century, made a remarkable recovery from a savage war wound to his stomach. The recovery left the man with some of the lining of his stomach outside his body: bizarre but true. What Pavlov noted was that whenever he became hungry, even before he began to eat, his now inside-out stomach put forth all sorts of digestive juices as he prepared for his *expected* feast. At dinner time his stomach poured. If he smelled food, it poured. In other words, his brain was somehow getting his stomach to work *before* the food arrived.

Pavlov operated on a dog to give him a similar inside-out piece of stomach and performed some experiments with his laboratory pet that made them both famous. In essence, after much work, Pavlov found that he could condition the dog so that he would make it pour out gastric juices when neither food nor hunger was involved.

If you take an animal such as Pavlov's dog and ring a loud bell every time you expose it to a delicious aroma that would normally get its juices flowing you can soon get those same juices flowing just by ringing the bell. Whatever message usually goes from the brain to the stomach with hunger now travels the same pathways when a bell is rung. This learned response is called conditioning.

So entrenched into the scientific soul of behavioural psychologists and physiologists is conditioning that it is not surprising that some of the first and most interesting attempts at demonstrating that the mind controls or at least can influence the immune system came from conditioning experiments. Let me give you a few examples.

If you take an ordinary mouse and inject into it some red blood cells from say, a sheep, the mouse's immune system will obviously object. Its T cells will recognise the intruders, sound the alarm, and among other things activate his B cells to make antibodies to the sheep's blood cells. Three weeks later you would not have trouble detecting these antibodies in a few drops of the mouse's blood. All perfectly normal.

Today we have drugs that poison B cells. We use them to treat diseases in which B cells are so disturbed that they become a menace, e.g., some forms of leukemia. Such a drug is cyclophosphamide, which we will call Cy for short. If you put Cy (which is tasteless) in the drinking water of our mouse and give him some sheep red blood cells, he will not make as much antibody as the mouse given plain water. After a couple of weeks the mouse given the Cy recovers and is back to normal. At this stage he would respond quite normally if given a second injection of sheep red blood cells.

Into such a model you can add a conditioning trick. Say you add some saccharin to the water as well as the Cy and then inject the sheep red blood cells. Now we know the water is very sweet, and, of course, the mouse still does not make as much antibody as normal because the Cy in the water poisons his B cells.

Allow the mouse to recover and repeat the sequence. Allow him to recover again but on a third, time only put saccharin in the water—no drugs. What do you think will happen to his antibody production? You are right. It is suppressed.

Saccharin will initiate a taste signal that goes to the brain where it is translated as 'it-must-be-B-cell-suppression-time'. That message in the brain leads to a chain of events that suppresses the B cell response and yet there is no poison in sight. Obviously the clever scientists doing these experiments had to show that saccharin *per se* had no effect on antibody production, and they did.

Encouraged by these remarkable observations, these sorts of experiments were varied. There is a mouse strain known as the NZB (New Zealand Black) mouse which is famous in the immunological world because it contracts systemic lupus erythematosus (SLE), almost identical to the strain humans get. After a few months of life, auto antibodies form in this strain of mouse and destroy many of his normal tissues including his red cells and kidneys. The disease can be prevented by giving the NZB mouse Cy from an early age. We now know that the same conditioning tricks described above allow saccharin to minimise the disease while subjecting the mouse to many fewer side effects than one would produce by continuing to treat him with Cy. You can see the potential use for this approach in humans.

This sort of evidence is not just restricted to experiments performed in this strain of mouse, nor to the use of saccharin. If you take a guinea pig, for example, and graft onto its side a small piece of rabbit skin, what happens?

Healthy guinea pig T cells recognise that the rabbit skin is foreign and in a few days attack in full force with millions of cells invading the rabbit's tissue and destroying it. If that experiment is done but an 'operation' of the operation is made, another example of conditioning is demonstrated, e.g. doing the skin graft while playing some music in the room and having differently colored lights flashing on and off. You give the animal an injection of local anesthetic in the area in which you will place the graft and then wrap up the site in big bandages that make it awkward for the guinea pig to walk. In other words, the guinea pig learns that lights, music, anesthetic and bandages are associated with the placement of a graft on his side.

If you do this three times, but on the third time you do not place any rabbit skin on the side of the animal, what happens? There is no skin to reject, of course, but if you biopsy the skin a week or so later, where the graft *would* have been you find the skin full of angry-looking T cells searching everywhere for a foreign graft that is expected to be present but is not. These little T cells obviously were given a message from the guinea pig's brain to expect trouble.

How could a guinea pig learn that lights, etc., mean that a skin graft was to be expected so that messages could be sent from its brain to its T cells urging that they be on the lookout for trouble in a specific area? The answers to such a riddle are not all in, but we are getting close as you will see.

If the mind can influence the immune system, could stress, in general, or perhaps a particular form of stress, damage the immune system of some animals and in this way produce a model for what may have happened to Martina?

The study of the way in which a genetic makeup may make one animal perform better under stressful conditions than another is fascinating. For most of these sorts of experiments we use small laboratory animals which we have inbred to the point where all the animals are identical. That is, we have hundreds of cloned animals all with an identical genetic makeup.

If you take a rat or a mouse and fix it in its cage so that it has little room to move and you strap electrodes to its tail, you can stress the animal for various periods by delivering very small electric shocks to its tail. The shock is tiny but obviously unpleasant.

Numerous such studies have shown that rats and mice become physically ill from this treatment, despite normal amounts of food and water. The physical deterioration noted involves a dramatic decrease in T cell function and a marked increase in susceptibility to infection. But isn't this all wrong? Shouldn't the stress get the animal fighting mad and ready for flight? Shouldn't the T cells be turned *on*, not off?

In some animals the reverse does happen. Certain strains of mice lose weight and hair lustre and have T cell depression for quite some time after the stress begins, but then they recover spontaneously. Their weight increases and their T cells become, in fact, super-efficient. They have adapted to the stress magnificently.

Other strains of mice, given a similar set of stressful circumstances, simply fade away. This obviously suggests that genetic information can help us perform better under stress. Most interestingly, preliminary studies seem to show that if you inject some serum from the mouse that has successfully adapted to a stressful situation into an inadequate mouse, the latter becomes a fighter. If this is confirmed, can you imagine how valuable will be the blood of the cool calm efficient IBM executive who thrives on the stress of his job?

The mouse that roared in the face of stress as described above (inescapable tail shock) is the exception rather than the rule, so it brings us back to the 'how come' question we asked before. Shouldn't stress improve physical responses if Darwin's fright and flight concepts are right?

Psychologists have long thought that the *deleterious* responses to stress that one may find associated with a certain set of circumstances can be markedly reduced if we have room to manoeuvre in the situation. If you can respond to the stressful situation in a positive fashion, in other words you can do something about the situation, the harmful effects of stress are reduced. Could the ability to cope with danger or, for that matter, with constant pain, etc., be the important factors that determine the effect of stress on the immune system?

Back to the laboratory we go and take two sets of identical rats. We place electrodes on their tails and intermittently shock them slightly at ten-second intervals for three minutes. Both sets get the same shock. One set of rats, however, have in their cage a small lever and when they learn to push this lever with their paw the shocks will stop. The shocks will also stop for the other group but they have no way of controlling the situation; they were not involved in actions that spared them pain.

It is amazing how quickly the rats with the levers in their cage will learn to turn off the shocks and, although stressed by having the shocks start all over again at variable intervals, the animals that can turn off the shocks thrive. Not so the rats who feel the same shocks but are helpless. They lose weight and have their immune system depressed.

Thus it would seem that for most of us, stress causes the brain to initiate a series of endocrine and immune responses that help us terminate the stress. Successful application of these moves with subsequent lessening of stress is called coping. If it so happens that circumstances make it impossible to handle the situation, many important systems in the body may not function normally and disease may result.

In this context it is important to realise that if circumstances are really impossible to handle or just *perceived* to be impossible to handle, the results may be the same. How much stress an individual human can handle without getting into trouble varies considerably, as it does with mice.

Before we talk about studies and observations of the interactions of the human mind and immune system we should look at possible ways that the interdependency of the nervous, endocrines and immune systems could occur. If the sensation of taste can pass from nerves in the tongue to the center of the brain, which appreciates taste, and then initiate effects that stop B cells in the spleen from making antibodies, then there must be brain-lymphocyte connections.

We are all used to thinking of the brain sending messages down nerves in the spinal cord which will branch off between the vertebrae to connect muscles and blood vessels, etc., to headquarters (the brain) in a physical fashion. You can follow the messages from initiation to reception.

Messages, of course, race back along similar pathways to tell the brain the desired effect has, or has not, occurred. If you move your toe right now you have sent a message at incredible speed to the muscles of your foot. This has resulted in your moving your toe and this results in the message being sent back to the brain so that, in fact, you know you have really moved your toe.

That system isn't good enough to connect the immune system to the brain, however, for, as we have seen when discussing our immune system, we are talking about collections of cells patrolling around the body; they are certainly not dancing on the ends of any nerves like puppets on a string.

The brain is composed of numerous subsections that control specific functions. Smell, speech, sight and hearing, for example, are all controlled by different parts of the brain. This is why it is possible for someone who has had a stroke (i.e., had damage occur to a small part of their brain by interference to that region's blood supply) to lose, say, the ability to speak while still being able to comprehend the written or spoken word.

It is possible for scientists who are trying to map the specific functions of various geographical areas of the brain to place a small electrode, via an extremely thin needle, into certain parts of the brain. The scientist may then send an electrical message through the electrode that will either stimulate that specific part of the brain or he may damage it and see what happens to the animal when this section of the brain is no longer working.

Studies on parts of the brain in humans can be so specific, for example, that stimulation of a specific area will always invoke the same memory. A specific memory circuit has obviously been located.

Using such techniques and others, scientists have studied areas of the brain which may influence the performance of the immune system. Already much has been learned. We know that nerves pass from the brainstem directly to the thymus gland in the neck. You remember the thymus is the immune system's 'soul'. These nerve fibres indicate that messages can pass from the brain to the thymus and vice versa. What sort of signals are dispatched along these newly discovered fibres is unknown but they are not there by chance—something important is going on.

There is a little gland in the brain called the pineal gland. It is very important in regulating sleep patterns and in regulating many other rhythms that fluctuate between night and day. Damage to this gland damages the ability of immunoregulatory T cells to do their job in a way that is as yet poorly understood.

Damage to the hypothalamus, which is so vital for the initiation of hormonal responses, also damages many aspects of immune function, inhibiting the ability of lymphocytes to circulate and regulate their own activity. In addition, those non-specific scavenger cells that mop up the immunological debris (dead bacteria, etc.) are prevented from performing normally by some as yet unknown mechanisms when the hypothalamus is damaged. If you damage the left side of the brain but not the right side you will damage natural killer cell (NK) activity.

In summary, we now know that the brain has many circuits that are linked in some way into the heart of the immune system. That leaves us with the problem of how the interaction occurs. Faced with this dilemma, scientists began to seek evidence that the mind that uses the ability to control the release of hormones could use them or another set of chemicals to deliver messages to the cells of the immune system.

For this to be possible, we would need to show that the wall of the lymphocyte, that is, its outer membrane, is equipped with the necessary receptors for accepting such chemical messages. There is no use having a lot of adrenalin, for example, arriving at the surface of the lymphocyte if the cell has no way of knowing that it is being bombarded with this hormone.

As you have no doubt guessed, the surface of lymphocytes turns out to be bristling with antennae for the reception of various hormones and chemicals. Lymphocytes have receptors for insulin, steroids, adrenalin and a host of other potent chemicals. But lymphocytes and other cells of the immune system themselves secrete chemicals and therefore could potentially send messages back to the brain (if the brain had nerve cells that could read these signals); of course it does. The science of psycho-neuroendocrinoimmunology is with us.

This extension of the concept that danger, etc., provokes not only neuroendocrine interactions but also neuroendocrine immunological re-actions would no doubt have delighted Darwin, who was so interested in the defense of man, but there are some potential traps in it for the human species.

I suspect that for centuries doctors have observed 'the fighting spirit phenomenon' and certainly many would tell you that depressed patients are more likely to suffer frequent infections. But suspecting this and proving this suspicion are two different things. Depressed patients may have more problems with infection if the depression itself depressed their immune system, but there could be simpler explanations. Depressed people do not eat as well as others; their standards of personal hygiene may slip. These factors may play a major role in producing health problems.

We are now certain that depression is associated with suppressed immunological functions in humans. Here we run into the difficulties that plague this sort of research; measuring in objective terms a degree of depression is much more difficult than documenting a specific percent-age decrease in T cell function. For this reason it is perhaps easiest for scientists interested in the question to study emotional extremes to find out if they are on the right track.

Perhaps the most potent emotion experienced by man is that sorrow which follows bereavement, the overwhelming sadness associated with the loss of someone loved. Characteristically this emotion is not short-lived and therefore such an intensive experience is indeed able to engender hormonal and/or immunological changes. One may expect that clinically significant results might occur. Panic can be even more dramatic than bereavement, of course, but it is so shortlived (you make it or you do not make it) that there may not be enough time for any significant change to occur.

Even when studying something as powerful as bereavement one must remember that while all intelligent species who can feel are subject to emotions associated with bereavement, in humans, and probably animals, there is a variation in the intensity of bereavement that is both cultural and individual. Most people are more or less devastated for four to six weeks after the loss of someone loved and then they pick up the pieces of their life and march on. Others take months or years to pull out of the depths of their depression, with disastrous results to their social and working lives.

Psychologists, of course, cannot specify an exact time for a normal grief response period, but in their analysis of the individual case they can decide that, yes, this person's suffering is beyond the normal, in fact it is pathological bereavement.

We are not going to discuss those pathological situations. What we will look at is the effect that bereavement, handled normally, has on the immune system of otherwise *healthy* individuals. That is, we will be looking at the sort of emotion you may see in a man who is grief-stricken for four to six weeks after his wife dies, who suffers episodic depression over a period of months as he faces life alone.

Statistical analysis of mortality figures tell us that men, at any age, who lose a wife, have a fourteen times greater chance of dying within the next twelve months than if they had not been so bereaved. What happens to them? Do they try and clean out the electric toaster while it is still plugged in? Do they fall and hit their heads in the parking lot of the supermarket on a snowy day? We do not know. The figures I quoted are just that; statistical facts which are now being carefully researched.

Some preliminary studies have reported that women have a threefold less chance of dying the year after their husbands die than if their husbands had survived. Psychologists argue that most women, either at a conscious or subconscious level expect that their husbands will die first, and if they do in fact die first, they are prepared—conditioned over the years.

Men never think that their wives will die first and the shock is therefore so much worse, especially if they are left with young children to rear. Studies have shown that suppression of the immune system after the loss of a wife is directly proportional to the troubles experienced in handling children now left without a mother.

Most of the studies of this scenario have been restrospective, which introduces problems. One does not really know that a person who is immunosuppressed after a loss has not developed his present problems because his immune system was not normal before bereavement. Secondly, historical details which are often sketchy, might be wrong. Therefore prospective studies are needed and these are indeed under way.

Some of the problems associated with the studies we are talking about can be overcome by looking at depression in animals. Bereavement can be induced in animals, and the effects studied. One model that has received a lot of attention creates a loss and then corrects the situation, thus allowing us to look not only at the effect of bereavement on the immune system, but also to repair mechanisms to the damage that has been done.

Monkeys are very emotional animals and have long been known to suffer physical changes while bereaved. Experiments which sound cruel (and are) but are of vital importance, involve the study of maternal deprivation among monkeys. Baby monkeys can be removed from their natural mothers at an early age and the effect of separation upon both mother and baby studied.

Various conditions can be established. The babies are sometimes given to other mothers who have or have not had their own baby monkeys removed so that some maternal care, if not the correct maternal care, can be supplied. Alternatively, the baby monkeys can be totally cared for by humans. After a period of studying monkeys deprived of their mothers the youngsters can be reunited with their natural mothers and the effects of this emotional reunion can be measured.

Studies have shown that maternally deprived monkeys become agitated over a two-week period and then become depressed, the latter being judged by disturbances in their sleep patterns and very decreased activity. Both mother and baby suffer a very significant deterioration in T cell function. Physically reuniting mothers and babies, however, very rapidly reverses the damage and by looking at the data there is little trouble in determining which babies had been returned to their mothers and which had not.

As you would probably expect, something like great sadness may cause the release of many hormones simultaneously and it does not necessarily follow that all the hormones released will affect the immune system. Mapping the hormonal changes associated with a particular emotion would be the first step to asking which hormone or hormones change the immune system. Scientists at New York's Mt Sinai hospital are studying this subject with the help of some remarkable people.

Even if the reader is not a parent, I am sure he or she can understand the particularly devastating sadness associated with *knowing* you are about to lose a child.

I have constantly observed over more than twenty years as a doctor that most people die with a degree of resignation that ensures dignity and speaks well of the basic human realism that can be brought to bear on this one inescapable occurrence. Children certainly are no exception, although they must face death within the limits of their intellectual development.

After explaining the nature of their research and its importance to parents who are about to lose a child, these doctors have invited their help by requesting that blood samples be constantly monitored before, during and after a near-final meeting with a dying child. A thin plastic catheter is placed in a vein in the arm so that blood can be withdrawn at will and unobtrusive electrodes are placed on the scalp so that brainwaves can be measured. From this type of research will come clues to how the brain and the body's chemicals interact with the immune system.

While we are examining connections between the brain and the immune system, we must not overlook an important but as yet poorly understood set of interactions involving lefthandedness. Medical and physical consequences are associated with this preference.

First, the good part. Among true lefties (that is, excluding ambidextrous people) there is a disproportionately high number who, because of a heightened appreciation of spatial concepts, are very good at such things as sport, the arts and architecture. In addition, there is a lack of the common mental illness schizophrenia among lefthanded people.

But the news is not all good. Left handed people have twelve times more learning disabilities than do righthanded people and stuttering and autism are more common. While lefties do not get schizophrenia they do seem to be more prone to suffer from manic-depressive psychosis, a severe problem that manifests itself as the blackest of depressions alternating with manic behaviour. There is a delusionary component to the illness so that the victim, for example, may feel very rich during his manic phase and race around the city buying thousands of dollars' worth of goods he does not need and certainly cannot afford.

In our context, however, we are interested in an association between lefthandedness and the early onset of childhood allergies and a number of autoimmune diseases such as ulcerative colitis, myasthenia gravis and coeliac disease.

So that I am not besieged with letters beginning 'I'm lefthanded and have never stuttered in my entire life,' let me stress that most lefthanded people have none of these problems (I also know a lot of terrible lefthanded tennis players). It is clear that lefthandedness *per se* is not the cause of these problems, though it may frequently be associated with other abnormalities that do cause problems.

When the embryonic brain is developing, some sections seem dependent for normal growth on the presence of more or less of the male sex hormone testosterone. If there is a little too much testosterone then an area of the brain known as the *planum temporale* overdevelops in the right hand section of the brain and the result is a 'lefty'.

As we discussed in the section on autoimmune disease, such problems are much more common among women than men and it may well be that an imbalance in sex hormone concentrations during fetal development causes not only lefthandedness, but the development of less than perfect central nervous system connections to the immune system. This may result in the loss of certain regulatory controls that normally prevent autoimmunity.

Summarising to this point, we can see that the immunological defense of man is in the hands of lymphocytes; cells that can be influenced by the central nervous system either directly, e.g., nervous innovation of the thymus, or indirectly by hormones controlled by the brain. Lymphocytes can also send messages to the brain so it is definitely a two way street. The potential for mental conditioning that might strengthen our defense mechanisms is obviously an exciting area for exploration, as is the possibility that higher center-generated feelings, such as depression, might damage the immune system of some. Let us look at both ideas but the latter first.

Let us visit the West Point Military Academy in New York state in any typical year, and take a look at the young candidates for officership who get glandular fever. The correct name of this disease, as we discussed earlier, is infectious mononucleosis, known as mono. It is a miserable disease and it is very infectious.

In a place like West Point it takes only one or two recruits to come down with the disease after picking up the virus and the whole academy is in trouble. Under dormitory conditions it is easy for the virus to spread and a mini-epidemic will result.

One of the interesting things about infectious mononucleosis is that not everyone infected with the virus that causes the disease suffers the same fate. Some have a very mild flulike illness, while others can be bedridden for six months or longer and even die of complications.

In some people in Africa the virus can trigger off a cancer in the immune system, while in Asia it can trigger a cancerous growth at the back of the nose and throat. A good immune system is certainly needed to handle this virus which in some respects is a close relative of the AIDS virus.

EBV belongs to a different family of viruses than the retrovirus that causes AIDS, but mono does result in an infection occurring within lymphocytes — B cells in this case, not T cells as in AIDS. We are then left with the distasteful task of killing our infected B cells and just how long it takes our T cells to do this job determines the length and severity of the disease. The point is that EBV virus infection is a great challenge for the immune system.

What would one find if one analysed both the clinical disease, i.e., how sick an individual becomes and the immune response to the virus, and related these findings to various psychosocial features that might be important at a place like West Point?

This training ground for young officers is full of cadets whose fathers were either graduates themselves or are professionals in the military forces. It seems, on careful examination, that a lot of the young students are only there because their fathers want them to be there. In such circumstances, many have a miserable time of it and do poorly in their examinations.

Studies showed a clear separation between those who made a very good immunological response to the virus once infected and those who did less well. Those students who were not happy at West Point and were under a considerable amount of stress because of doubts about their career choice had more symptoms and their immunological response to the disease was poor. There was an equally strong correlation between satisfaction with the establishment and a good response to the infectious agent.

I can give you many other examples, but two will suffice. You will remember we mentioned NK or natural killer cells. These are the cells that spontaneously attack malignant cells that may appear in the body and destroy them.

Their action is almost immediate and there seems no reason to imagine that these cells do not play an important role on a day-to-day basis in protecting us from the development of cancer. Their action depends on the presence in the body of the naturally occurring chemical interferon.

We have known for some time that a number of potential cancer-causing chemicals depress NK cell activity and the depressed NK cell activity is associated with increased risk of getting cancer. More recently we have learned that NK cells performance is very markedly affected by stress. When these cells are activated by interferon, they become somewhat larger-than-normal lymphocytes and have a granular appearance that makes them easy to recognise. Recently a number of scientists involved in behavioural immunology have begun to call them 'stress lymphocytes'.

Studies have been done among medical students at Johns Hopkins University while undergoing stressful examinations. It certainly would appear as though those candidates who were less well prepared for their examinations and who subsequently did poorly were under a lot of stress. Their stress and failure correlated very well with depressed NK cell activity. These studies are particularly interesting because they suggest once again that the nature of the stressful event and one's ability to cope with that stress determine whether one's immune system performs adequately.

One final example of this sort of thing comes from dental students who are having examinations. Here it was found that those students who were suffering from a great deal of stress because they were less well prepared for the examinations did poorly in their exams, as would be expected. They also had an increased occurrence of upper respiratory tract infections following those exams. No such effects, of course, were noted in those students who did well and who were well prepared for the exams.

What was so fascinating to these particular observers was the fact that secretory IgA, the specific immunoglobulin that protects our mucous membranes and therefore our upper airways, was suppressed in those students experiencing much stress at exam time. It is entirely feasible to suggest that the suppression of this form of antibody response left them vulnerable to upper respiratory tract infections.

A little earlier I mentioned that, apart from the potentially harmful effects of stress on the immune system that clinicians will have to deal with in the future, it was also necessary to contemplate the possibility of *improving* immunological responses by conditioning. Some very encouraging results have been reported recently.

If you remember our little mouse taking the saccharin and how he could be tricked into suppressing his immune system with just a sweetener, then you can understand why it is that clinicians may want to use conditioning approaches to improve a person's immune response to his own cancer.

Scientists in the United States used this approach with a group of doctors suffering from cancer. These doctors were ideal candidates for this form of experimentation because they had elected not to receive any conventional treatment for their cancer. Let me hasten to add that these were not in any way a group of anti-medical establishment doctors who were seeking alternative medicine approaches to their cancer; far from it. These were doctors, who because of their lifelong experience in the profession knew that the cancer from which they suffered meant that they had at best a few extra months to be gained by submitting themselves to chemotherapy. In their minds, any suppression of the cancer would be more than offset by the loss of the quality of their life caused by the side effects of the drugs that would be required. For such physicians the chance to take part in conditioning exercises was most appealing.

The physicians were first educated about their immune system as many of them would certainly not have kept up with the more recent information about immunology that we have been discussing in this book. It was explained to them that they did have immune cells with the capacity to kill tumor cells if only they could be activated to do so. They were shown slides and movie films of normal cells killing tumor cells in a test tube and were asked to concentrate on sending signals from the brain to the immune system demanding that similar proficiency be developed for the fight against their own cancer.

The physicians had immunological studies done before their conditioning experiments started and, among the immune function studies performed were ones to look at their ability to kill cancer cells. Needless to say, the studies were repeated during and after the conditioning therapy.

While it is too early to determine whether these particular doctors had their life prolonged significantly by these conditioning experiments (the final results have not been reported in the literature) the preliminary reports clearly demonstrated that these physicians were able to increase the cancer-fighting capacity of their immune system.

A more extensive trial for this sort of work is under way at the M.D. Anderson Cancer Center in Texas. Again, while the results are preliminary, the initial impressions of the investigators have been very favorable. In this study, it seems that there is a correlation between increased activity against tumor cells and a longer than expected survival time.

Numerous other pieces of the psychoimmunology jigsaw puzzle are being reported and need further investigating. There is at least a twofold greater incidence of cancer among humans who suffer a long period of depression after loss or separation. There is a particular risk, for example, that men in that situation may develop testicular cancer. Juvenile rheumatoid arthritis, an immunological attack on the joints of children, is much more common among adopted children and children who have suffered through a traumatic divorce.

Other investigators have reported that children who grow up in a household where they feel that there is a lack of closeness have a much higher risk of developing cancer later in life. Autistic children who appear to have withdrawn from the world clearly have depressed T cell function. We can go on and on but I feel that this review has given you the flavor for one of the most exciting areas of modern medicine.

In closing, we must stress that although there is voluminous literature on the subject, there are few really good scientific studies that have been carried out with all the safeguards that top class scientists would demand. These are under way and there seems little doubt that information of great value will be available to us in the next few years.

In the meantime, it is probably wise for all of us to think carefully about the words of wisdom provided by the American cardiologist Robert Elliot. In worrying about type A personalities (whose anxiety and pace of life may lead to early heart attack), he promulgated two useful rules. Rule 1 was: don't sweat the small stuff. Very good advice.

But Rule 2 is even more useful. This rule simply states: 'It's all small stuff'.

Certainly, we can extend the concepts important in controlling heart disease to the control of those diseases linked to abnormal functioning of the immune and endocrine systems. Perhaps, therefore, we will leave the subject with some famous reflections on behavioural immunology from that well-known observer of the human scene Mr Woody Allen. Trotting forth his wisdom in the movie *Manhattan*, he supplies the following lines which clearly demonstrate his knowledge of psycho-neuro-immunology.

'Well, I don't get angry, O.K.

I mean, I have a tendency to internalise.

I can't express anger.

That's one of the problems I have.

I—I grow a tumor instead.'

Index